MENTAL ILLNESS

Recent Titles in
Health and Medical Issues Today

Obesity
Evelyn B. Kelly

Organ Transplantation
David Petechuk

Stem Cells
Evelyn B. Kelly

Alternative Medicine
Christine A. Larson

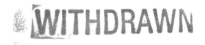
MENTAL ILLNESS

Marie L. Thompson

Health and Medical Issues Today

GP

GREENWOOD PRESS
Westport, Connecticut • London

Library of Congress Cataloging-in-Publication Data

Thompson, Marie L., 1947–
   Mental illness / Marie L. Thompson.
      p.   cm. — (Health and medical issues today, ISSN 1558–7592)
   Includes bibliographical references and index.
   ISBN 0–313–33565–6 (alk. paper)
      1. Mental illness—Popular works.   I. Title.
   RC460.T46   2007
   618.89—dc22   2006028663

British Library Cataloguing in Publication Data is available.

Library of Congress Catalog Card Number: 2006028663
ISBN: 0–313–33565–6
ISSN: 1558–7592

First published in 2007

Greenwood Press, 88 Post Road West, Westport, CT 06881
An imprint of Greenwood Publishing Group, Inc.
www.greenwood.com

Printed in the United States of America

The paper used in this book complies with the
Permanent Paper Standard issued by the National
Information Standards Organization (Z39.48–1984).

10   9   8   7   6   5   4   3   2   1

CONTENTS

SERIES FOREWORD

Every day, the public is bombarded with information on developments in medicine and health care. Whether it is on the latest techniques in treatments or research, or on concerns over public health threats, this information directly impacts the lives of people more than almost any other issue. Although there are many sources for understanding these topics—from Web sites and blogs to newspapers and magazines—students and ordinary citizens often need one resource that makes sense of the complex health and medical issues affecting their daily lives.

The *Health and Medical Issues Today* series provides just such a one-stop resource for obtaining a solid overview of the most controversial areas of health care today. Each volume addresses one topic and provides a balanced summary of what is known. These volumes provide an excellent first step for students and lay people interested in understanding how health care works in our society today.

Each volume is broken into several sections to provide readers and researchers with easy access to the information they need:

- Section I provides overview chapters on background information—including chapters on such areas as the historical, scientific, medical, social, and legal issues involved—that a citizen needs to intelligently understand the topic.
- Section II provides capsule examinations of the most heated contemporary issues and debates, and analyzes in a balanced manner the viewpoints held by various advocates in the debates.

- Section III provides a selection of reference material, including annotated primary source documents, a timeline of important events, and an annotated bibliography of useful print and electronic resources that serve as the best next step in learning about the topic at hand.

The *Health and Medical Issues Today* series strives to provide readers with all the information needed to begin making sense of some of the most important debates going on in the world today. The series will include volumes on such topics as stem-cell research, obesity, gene therapy, alternative medicine, organ transplantation, mental health, and more.

PREFACE

Mental illness as understood by the modern biomedical model is highly prevalent worldwide. In the United States, it affects approximately 22 percent of the population, including children and adolescents, in any given year. More than half of all adults will experience some form of mental illness at some time in their life. Globally, mental illness ranks second only to cardiovascular disease on the burden of disease scale.

Mental illness has a history at least as long as recorded history. It also has a history of misunderstanding, stigma, and discrimination, all of which are still significantly present even in well-educated societies and all of which can be reduced by information and education. This book provides a very basic overview of a huge and complex subject with the aim of providing awareness and thought-provoking topics for the reader to research further. The first section depicts how mental illness has been perceived and treated throughout the ages, defines the modern biomedical model, presents statistical information on its prevalence, and traces the evolution of psychology and of twentieth-century scientific research, diagnostic methods and criteria, and treatment modalities. The second section introduces some important controversies: perspectives that strongly dispute the biomedical model, that criticize the field of psychiatry, and some that even deny the very existence of mental illness; issues surrounding treatment safety and efficacy and drug company ethics; civil liberty issues pertaining to involuntary commitment and outpatient treatment; the process of deinstitutionalization and the corresponding increase in incarceration and homeless rates; insurance disparity; the dilemma of maintaining patient confidentiality; legal and political acts and their consequences; and legal processes involved in crimes committed by the mentally ill. The book in its entirety presents a concise overview of mental illness and of both sides of these controversial related issues. The bibliography contains sources of information gathered for compilation of the book, most of which are readily accessible on the Internet and which contain a wealth of information that can barely be touched on in this limited volume. Because the book is intended to increase awareness and understanding of issues surrounding mental illness and, as such, to contribute to continuing efforts to eliminate discrimination, stigma, and misunderstanding, it is hoped that the reader will access these Web sites and that those with a mental health issue will utilize the listed resources to become better informed and develop a deeper insight into the complicated controversies surrounding mental illness.

INTRODUCTION

Throughout history, people with certain behavioral and emotional traits have been recognized by the societies in which they lived as differing significantly from the general population. Attitudes toward and treatment of those unique individuals varied between cultures and changed over time. Some cultures believed such individuals were overtaken by spirits that could be either good or evil; some believed their "strange" behavior was caused by inner conflict because of their sins; some believed it was a gift from God; some believed it was possession by the devil. Some ancient Arabs, Greeks, and Romans had insights into causes and treatment methods amazingly similar to certain treatments proposed by twenty-first-century psychiatry. Historically, those suffering from what was once called lunacy or madness and is now known as mental illness or mental disorder have variously been treated kindly and cruelly. Even in the twenty-first century—with medical, scientific, and psychiatric researchers working diligently to understand causes and develop effective treatments for mental illness—misconception, misunderstanding, and mystery still surround the subject.

The twentieth century brought with it the development of amazing advances and achievements in research, technology, medicine, neurosciences, and psychiatry. By midcentury, psychiatry and psychoanalysis was in full swing, and literally hundreds of psychotherapeutic methods evolved. The 1950s saw the introduction of the first reference manual to assist physicians in diagnosing mental illnesses. It was also the dawning of the clinical application of psychotropic drugs, and early excitement about their efficacy led many to believe, incorrectly, that they would actually cure mental illness. In 1953, the structure and properties of DNA—the blueprint of life—was revealed, and a decade or so later, imaging techniques opened a window into the brain. Researchers studied neuro-transmitters, their role in communication between neurons in the brain, and their mechanisms of action—gathering significant evidence that too much or too little of certain of these brain chemicals caused certain mood or behavioral disorders. In the 1990s, "new-generation" antidepressant and "atypical" antipsychotic medications became available for treating depression and schizophrenia, respectively, supposedly with fewer and less troublesome side effects. Advances in imaging techniques enabled three-dimensional, full-color images of the brain from different viewing planes to be constructed, and by the close of the century, neuroscientists had a plethora of evidence linking different physical and emotional functions to different areas in the brain.

By the early twenty-first century, approximately 99 percent of the human genome had been sequenced to a 99.99 percent accuracy—the fullest extent to which available technology would allow—and functional imaging techniques permitted visualization of the brain as it thinks and responds to stimuli. Researchers, scientists, and psychiatrists alike remained highly optimistic that further developments in some or all of those areas would bring them closer to solving the mystery of what causes mental illnesses: biological testing or brain imaging would provide defin-itive diagnoses; identification of specific genes associated with specific mental disorders would allow development of highly targeted drugs; con-tinued research would lead to methods of prevention and perhaps even cures for mental illnesses. Yet those goals have proven elusive, and regardless of whether mental illness is becoming more prevalent, as some suggest, or is being better or more frequently diagnosed, as others suggest, its incidence worldwide is increasing. The task ahead for all involved in the pursuit of understanding and treating mental illness remains exciting yet daunting.

The barriers faced by many who suffer from mental illnesses also remain daunting. Psychiatric institutionalization was too often and too long used as a means to remove the socially undesirable from society; to retain indefinitely against their will people who were able to function well in the community; to allow abuse, neglect, and forced treatments of all kinds; and to ruin and end many lives. Yet the deinstitutionalization that began with the advent of psychotropic drugs and continues to this day brought with it a different dilemma: it has created hundreds of thousands of homeless and vulnerable mentally ill and has criminalized hundreds of thousands more. Although millions of mental health consumers have experienced extremely beneficial—and in many cases, lifesaving—effects from available therapeutic methods, millions of others have not. Still others have been harmed by them, and some have died because of them.

The dilemma of treatment versus nontreatment is huge. Most people who know they have a mental illness remain untreated for various reasons, and national and international surveys have exposed the enormous psychological, physical, emotional, and financial burden of untreated mental illness to those who have it, to their families, and to society. Many advocates for the mentally ill demand that treatment be made more readily accessible—through avenues such as insurance parity and better-funded federal, state, and local governmental community health services. There are also those who believe treatment should be administered by court order when an individual diagnosed as seriously mentally ill refuses treatment or is too ill to either realize the need for treatment or cannot regulate his or her own treatment regimen. A primary reason for nontreatment is the stigma that surrounds mental illness. Stigma leads to discrimination, which often leads to a mentally ill individual being unable to obtain gainful employment or being fired. It also causes insurance inequity and lack of understanding of the plight of the mentally ill by much of society. Another reason for nontreatment is cost: treatment of any kind is expensive, and often prohibitively so, particularly for the seriously and persistently mentally ill who are usually unable to work.

On an even more fundamental level, the modern biomedical model of mental illness is vigorously opposed by "antipsychiatry" organizations and other groups that are not necessarily antipsychiatry but that nonetheless abhor many aspects of mainstream psychiatry due to what they deem to be its continuing misuse. Philosophies between these organizations can differ considerably: some highly trained psychiatrists dispute the very existence of mental illness and declare, therefore, that diagnosis and treatment are nothing but a farce; others call psychiatry a pseudoscience because it diagnoses mental illnesses when there is no concrete, definitive, scientific diagnostic method by which to do so; still others deem that treatment of any kind is detrimental, dangerous, and damaging; yet others maintain that psychiatry as an industry largely diagnoses individuals who display certain behavioral traits or nonconformist attitudes as being mentally ill and uses that diagnosis as either a means of social or political control or of maintaining an income stream for providers in the psychiatric industry. Almost all of these groups agree on one issue: they adamantly oppose the use of coercive (forced) institutionalization and outpatient treatment, and advocacy groups nationally and internationally fight for the civil liberties and human rights of people abused, neglected, and unlawfully retained in the name of psychiatry.

Scientific research continues its search for causes of and cures for mental illnesses, legal and political acts are proposed by supporters on both sides to deal with the many issues surrounding it, and moral and ethical debates pertaining to treatment and mistreatment of those diagnosed with it abound. An introduction to the complex and controversial subjects is presented in the following chapters, with the intention of bringing the educated lay reader some insight into these issues, of helping reduce stigma and discrimination, and of providing resources for mental health consumers and their families so that they, too, may better understand the nature of what is called mental illness and their options for dealing with it.

SECTION ONE

Background of Mental Illness

CHAPTER 1

What Is Mental Illness?

If society assumes that mind and brain are separate and that mental disorders are "different" or "bad," misunderstanding, mistreatment, and stigma will persist. If we see people as categories (e.g., schizophrenics, depressives), we will not see them as people.

Nancy C. Andreasen, *Brave New Brain: Conquering Mental Illness in the Era of the Genome*

From the beginning of recorded history, and probably from the beginning of human history, people have struggled to understand and explain mental illness. Even in the early twenty-first century, mental illness, along with the myriad of issues involved with it, remains a highly controversial topic. One school of thought maintains that mental illness does not exist, a rationale for that belief being that perceptions of the "norm" vary widely between and within cultures, and even between individuals. Therefore, what may be called mental illness by one culture or person may be regarded as quite natural behavior by another.

DEFINING MENTAL ILLNESS IN THE TWENTY-FIRST CENTURY

Mental illness is difficult to define, and the determination of what constitutes a mental illness changes over time. In 1968, for example, homosexuality, which is now considered by mainstream practice to be within the normal range of variation, was included in the second revision of the *Diagnostic and Statistic Manual of Mental Disorders* (DSM-II), the reference manual first published in 1952 by the American Psychiatric Associaton (APA), in which mental disorders are defined and diagnostic guidelines are presented. Not until 1973 did the APA vote to remove homosexuality from the manual.

The term *mental illness*, or *mental disorders*, as generally used in Western cultures, encompasses a large, and ever-evolving, number of diagnoses. Although some argue that the mind cannot become ill, the theory that mental illnesses are as real as physical illnesses is widely accepted. Whereas physical illnesses manifest in the body, mental illnesses manifest as certain types of behavior. Unlike physical illnesses, mental illnesses cannot be diagnosed by biological tests, such as viewing a virus under a microscope, imaging the brain, or doing blood tests. The exact origins of mental disorders remain elusive; however, many researchers and scientists believe they arise from some physical occurrence in the brain caused by psychological, biological, genetic, or environmental factors, or from some combination of such factors.

What Is It? What Is It Not?

The National Association for the Mentally Ill (NAMI) defines mental illness as "disorders [that] can profoundly disrupt a person's thinking, feeling, moods, ability to relate to others and capacity for coping with the demands of life." The landmark analysis of mental illness by the U.S. surgeon general in 1999, *Mental Health: Report of the Surgeon General*, states that it is "the term that refers collectively to all diagnosable mental disorders. Mental disorders are health conditions that are characterized by alterations in thinking, mood, or behavior (or some combination thereof) associated with distress and/or impaired functioning." Mental health, on the other hand, is defined as "the successful performance of mental function, resulting in productive activities, fulfilling relationships with other people, and the ability to adapt to change and to cope with adversity. . . . mental health is the springboard of thinking and communication skills, learning, emotional growth, resilience and self-esteem."

Mental illness does not indicate weakness, lack of intelligence, or a defective character. It is not caused by poor upbringing, although environmental factors such as this often play a role. It affects people of all social, economic, geographic, age, gender, religious, and occupational groups. In the United States, women, African Americans, the young, the elderly, and the poor are at highest risk, but no identifiable group is exempt from it. An individual may experience mental illness over many years or over an entire lifetime, or symptoms may only develop later in life. The symptoms, their duration, and their intensity vary. Some individuals experience episodes of more extreme and less extreme symptoms; for some, symptoms go into remission; for others, symptoms are continuous. People with mild symptoms may function well without professional help, whereas those with more severe symptoms require professional treatment and often hospitalization. Some mental illnesses are intractable (particularly resistant to treatment); a great many more respond exceptionally well to treatment, with between 70 and 90 percent of treated individuals experiencing a significantly improved quality of life.

Mental illness cannot be viewed in isolation from physical functioning; the two are inseparable. Memory and cognition are mental functions, but because they are initiated in the brain, they are also physical functions. A change in brain chemistry—a physical occurrence, caused, perhaps, by something as seemingly benign as stress—can cause changes in mental functions that manifest as anxiety, panic attacks, or depression. Physical and mental are two inseparable components of the complete human experience. In attempting to understand the complexities of mental illness, it is important to understand that physical and mental, that is, body and mind, cannot exist in isolation from one another.

HISTORIC PERSPECTIVES

The Beginning

In prehistory, mental illness was perceived as coming from supernatural, magical spirits that disrupted the mind. Shamans performed rituals, conjured up spells, and used mind-altering drugs in an attempt to communicate with or to exorcise those spirits. Archeological evidence shows that Stone Age people even developed a crude form of surgery, possibly with the intent of curing mental illness, in which a hole was drilled through the afflicted person's skull, apparently to release the evil spirit trapped within (Figure 1.1). Evidence of this practice, called *trepanning*, is found in fossils of human skulls in South America and Europe dating back to 10,000 BC. The fact that new bone grew to cover the hole in some skulls indicates that patients had a surprisingly high survival rate.

Throughout history, mental illness has been misunderstood, feared, and stigmatized. Different civilizations in different parts of the world during different eras had their own concepts of what caused mental illness and struggled with how, or whether, to treat it. Like their Stone Age predecessors, ancient Egyptians (beginning about 3000 or 2000 BC) believed it to be magical in origin, but their belief in life after death added a religious dimension. Their society was highly conscious of the self—not just of the physical being, but also of the spiritual being that was thought to live to eternity. No distinction was made between mental and physical illnesses. All illness was attributed to physical causes (for example, they believed

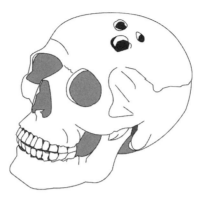

Figure 1.1
Trepanning in precivilization societies may have been attempts to release evil spirits believed to cause mental illness. (Ricochet Productions.)

the heart caused mental disturbances), to demonic possession, or to situations that angered one of their many gods, such as taboo violation or failure to perform ritual obligations. Both mind and soul were important to overall health in this belief system, and thus, by around the thirtieth century BC, a magical-religious concept of mental illness had developed that would ultimately last several thousand years and span many cultures.

The ancient Egyptians appear to have been the first to practice a form of mental health care. They developed the first known mental hospitals in temples and temple complexes and wrote the first known psychiatric text, and an ancient Egyptian was the first known physician to treat the mentally ill. Treatment consisted of rites, rituals, and prayers to specific gods; dream interpretation; and the use of opium to induce visions. Later, during the early Egyptian period, the loss of status or money was said to be the trigger of mental illness, and recommended treatments were based on a type of talk therapy in which patients were encouraged to turn to religion and faith.

The Influence of Monotheism: Judaism and Islam

Monotheism, the concept of one god, brought the next significant development in society's attitude toward mental illness. Although Israeli tribes can be traced back to approximately 2000 BC, Judaism underwent a significant growth period during the sixth century BC, when it began to be unified and organized. During this process, the concept of mental illness in Jewish society shifted away from the magical-religious into the realm of organized religion. Mental illness was viewed as the visible expression of sin, conflict in one's personal relationship with God, and of subsequent possession by demons. Treatment ranged from prayer and fasting to public self-flagellation (whipping) as repentance and penance. As portrayed by the Old Testament story of Job, the cause of mental illness was despair, and the cure was faith.

Also by the sixth century BC, Islam was well entrenched in Arabia and had begun to spread into Asia and Africa. Islam taught that people could come close to God only through radical changes in the way they perceived the universe. Mental illness was seen as a supernatural intervention in that process, a possession by *jinn*, or spirits, which could be either good or bad. This belief freed the concept of mental illness from those of sinfulness and demonic possession, and the causes of mental illness gradually came to be examined in a more scientific manner in Islamic society. Because the Arabs had no fear of demons, their patients were treated humanely. In Europe, however, where belief in demonic possession persisted, treatment facilities did not exist because people feared becoming possessed simply by associating with the mentally ill. Centuries later, the Islamic concept would dramatically influence Greek and European philosophies on mental illness.

Ancient Greek and Roman Philosophies

Ancient Greeks   Initially, the ancient Greeks perceived mental illness as stemming from the supernatural: Homer (c. 1200 BC) believed that God had taken away a mentally ill person's mind and that there was no cure; Aeschylus (525–456 BC) attributed mental illness to demonic possession and recommended exorcism; Socrates (469–399 BC) believed it to be a gift from God and thus a blessing that required no treatment.

Hippocrates (460–377 BC) presented a radical and amazingly insightful theory. He proposed that biological, or somatic, influences affected the brain, and he declared that "madness" was attributable to an imbalance of the four bodily humors, or fluids: blood, phlegm, and yellow and black bile. For example, he believed that black bile (*melan chole* in Greek) caused melancholia (sadness), now known as depression. He also described what are now known as mania, phobias, paranoia, and postpartum psychosis. His concept allowed for the idea that mental illness could be treated effectively, and he recommended therapy that would restore balance between the humors, which would rebalance the body, which would in turn rebalance the mind. Treatment included exercise, powders made from the leaves and roots of certain plants, a vegetarian diet, and abstinence from sex.

Although Hippocrates' ideas were not scientifically accurate, his theory of biological causes of mental illness is the foundation of the modern medical model. Certain disciplines falling under this model, such as Chinese medicine, still treat certain mental illnesses with herbs, natural substances, acupuncture, relaxation, and meditation. Western medicine has replaced the more natural treatments with treatment by psychotropic drugs and, less commonly, psychosurgery (operating on certain areas of the brain) and electroconvulsive therapy, or ECT (in which an electrical current is delivered to the brain).

Plato (428–348 BC) presented another theory that was brilliant for the era: that the mind itself caused madness and that ignorance of one's *psyche* (the human life force, or soul, and the Greek word from which the modern English word *psychology* is derived) led to self-deception and, subsequently, mental instability. His concept was of the *psyche* as a charioteer struggling to balance the conflicting desires of two powerful horses—one noble, the other ignoble. Plato's theory introduced the psychological perspective, a perspective similar to the superego, ego, and id of the famous nineteenth-century psychiatrist Sigmund Freud.

Aristotle (384–322 BC) proposed the importance of genetic inheritance, a theory undergoing considerable scientific study in the twenty-first century. He also believed that thoughts, feelings, and actions were intricately linked, and suggested a view of the mind that focused on its total interaction with the body, rather than one that separated individual faculties. The ancient Greeks therefore developed both mind and body theories of mental illness; however, the two schools of thought would remain independent until some attempts at unification were made in the early thirteenth century.

Ancient Romans   Although the ancient Greek concepts of mind were largely adopted by the ancient Romans, Hippocrates' biologically based theory was overshadowed by the supernatural and psychological perspectives. Cicero (106–143 BC), for one, rejected Hippocrates' biological theory and blamed mental illness on emotional disturbances. He proposed what may well be the most important early psychological theory pertaining to mental illness, suggesting that excessive "perturbations" (disturbances) of the mind cause diseases of the *psyche*. He observed that anxiety-prone people suffered from excessive perturbations and that a healthy soul required balance and harmony between its rational, irrational, and lustful aspects. He developed an assessment tool in the form of an interview that addressed social and personal issues, such as clan, family status, social class, education, passions, and significant life events. The tool was used throughout the Roman Empire and, indeed, by the Celtic monasteries until their dissolution in the 1500s. Cicero believed that people could cure their mental illnesses with philosophy, an idea that can be likened to modern-day psychotherapy.

This and other more enlightened concepts from Roman physicians were challenged in the last years before Christ. Cornelius Celsus (25 BC–AD 50) reintroduced the idea that angered gods caused some mental illnesses and recommended treatment such as restraint in chains, starvation, and whipping—anything "which thoroughly agitates the spirit." However, in a more scientific observation, the Roman medical philosopher Aretaeus (AD 50–130) accurately perceived that an individual could experience both manic and depressive states, with intervening periods of lucidity. He also recognized that mental illness did not necessarily equate with mental deterioration—a concept that was not well accepted even at the beginning of the twentieth century.

Middle Ages

During the early and High Middle Ages (500–1350), attempts were made to revive the Hippocratic theory. Constantinus Africanus (1020–1087), a Jew who converted to Christianity and who founded in Salerno, Italy, what is believed to be the world's first medical school, translated Hippocrates from Arabic into Latin and reintroduced the theory that mental illness arose in the brain. Attempts were also made to integrate the mind and body theories. Albert the Great (1206–1280) and Thomas Aquinas (1225–1274) presented significant psychological theories, their primary hypothesis being that the soul could not become sick and therefore somatic disturbances must cause insanity.

However, belief in supernatural causes remained strong. The Catholic Church began to dominate Europe both politically and socially shortly after the fall of the Roman Empire. Mental illness was perceived as a spiritual disturbance, and the church assumed authority over the afflicted. Challenging the church's doctrine concerning the origins of mental illness was deemed heretical: the Roman Catholic Inquisition, a tribunal instituted in Rome by Pope Innocent III (1160–1216) to interrogate and punish suspected heretics, ordered Pietro Albano (1250–1316) burned to death for minimizing spiritual philosophy while trying to align Aristotle's beliefs with medical facts about mental illness.

The late Middle Ages (1350–1500) was a disastrous era for the mentally ill. They became victims of persecution, and they were blamed for their own illness, accused of moral weakness, thought to be possessed by evil spirits, accused of indulging in forbidden associations with the devil, and expected to effect their own cure. Due to the rampant belief throughout Europe in witchcraft, many mentally ill people were accused of being witches possessed by demons. At first, the church made a distinction between involuntary and voluntary possession. Involuntary possession was perceived as punishment for sins, and priests used exorcisms and curses, prayer, and laying-on of hands, to dispel the devil. Voluntary possession was deemed to be the result of a conscious and deliberate pact with the devil for self-gain, and individuals who were thought to have made such a pact were branded as witches to be hanged, burned at the stake, or drowned.

Despite the widespread witch-hunt mentality of the sixteenth-century, there were some enlightened advocates for the mentally ill, such as Juan Luis Vives. Born in 1492 in Valencia, Spain, Vives was highly regarded by England's King Henry VIII as well as by Renaissance England's author and Catholic martyr St. Thomas More. He wrote considerably on issues pertaining to poverty and insanity, including the following words:

Now let us refer to the insane. Since there is nothing in the world more excellent than man, and nothing more excellent in man than his mind, particular care should be given to its welfare. It should be considered the highest of ministries to restore the mind of others to sanity, or to keep them sane and rational . . . One ought to feel a compassion before such a great disaster to this noblest of human faculties. He who has suffered so should be treated with such care and delicacy that the cure will not enlarge or increase the condition, such as would result from mocking, exciting, or irritating him, approving and applauding the foolish things which he says or does, and inciting him to act more ridiculously, applying a stimulus, as it were, to his absurdity and stupidity. What could be more inhumane than to drive a man to insanity just for the sake of laughing at him and entertaining oneself with such a misfortune!

Seventeenth through Nineteenth Centuries

From Witch Hunts to Lunatics By the 1600s, the division between voluntary and involuntary possession had become blurry, and many more mentally ill people were being branded as witches. This was particularly true of women. Demonic possession was perceived as the cause of mental illness, and women who suffered from it were accused of having copulated with the devil. A disproportionate number of women were thus put to death. In 1692 in Salem, Massachusetts, alone, nineteen people were tried and hanged for practicing witchcraft, fourteen of whom were women. During the 1500s and 1600s, many physicians challenged church doctrine, attempted to institute a more modern version of

Hippocrates' medical model, and tried to convince authorities that afflicted people were not insane but ill and needed appropriate care. These advocates were ridiculed and were often in danger of losing their practices and even their lives.

Not until the early 1700s did the supernatural explanation for mental illness shift. The mentally ill became known as lunatics and were perceived and treated as wild animals. Until the 1700s, they were usually cared for at home by their families, most often locked away in basements or attics for years or for their entire lives. Then the practice of institutionalization began. No distinction was made between the mentally ill and the criminally insane, and thousands of mentally ill—particularly the poor—were locked up in prisons with violent criminals in dark, dank cells, often unmercifully chained to the walls. Thousands more were sent to government welfare poorhouses (lunatic asylums), which were being established to house them. In either case, although the inmates received very basic care, conditions were appallingly overcrowded and unsanitary. Treatment consisted primarily of intimidation, physical abuse, and restraint in order to subdue the wild spirit within; the mortality rate was high. One of the most famous, or infamous, of these institutions was St. Mary of Bethlehem in London, England, commonly known as Bedlam—a name that has long since been used as a term to describe uproar or confusion. Some monasteries, however, offered more humane care, with rest, good food, occupational therapy, specially chosen music, and sleep, and gentle restraint for the agitated.

Signs of Reform In America in 1724, the Puritan clergyman Cotton Mather defied the perspective arising from superstition and advocated physical causes for mental illness. As the eighteenth century progressed, a more humanistic approach took shape. The first American hospital to accept mentally ill patients was the Pennsylvania Hospital, founded by the Quakers in 1751, where patients were kept—often locked and chained—in the basement. It was there that Benjamin Rush, a member of the medical staff for 29 years, began instituting reforms. Rush outlawed the use of whips, straitjackets, and chains, and, rather than simply lock people away, recommended treatment. Although many of his "treatment" methods, which included bloodletting, were controversial in their time and are considered harsh and barbaric by twenty-first-century standards, they were at least a step forward. Rush was also a professor at the Public Hospital for Persons of Insane and Disordered Minds, America's first psychiatric hospital. Located in Williamsburg, Virginia, it opened in 1773 and remained the only institution of its kind in America for the next 50 years.

Benjamin Rush (1745–1813) became known as the Father of American Psychiatry. Why is not clear, as the practice of psychiatry did not exist during his lifetime. It may be because of his lengthy study of mental illness and his treatise titled *Medical Inquires and Observations upon the Diseases of the Mind*. Published in 1812, this was the first—and for many years the only—treatise on mental illness in America. Rush developed the theory that disordered blood flow and inflammation of the brain caused mental illness. He advocated bloodletting, as well as purging by forced vomiting, to subdue the more violent patients. He also created mechanical devices intended to calm the patient and to direct blood flow to the brain. One device, the gyrator, acted like a spoke in a wheel. The patient was strapped supine to a board, and the contraption was spun to increase the patient's pulse rate and force blood to the brain. Another device was the tranquilizer chair, in which the patient was bound and unable to move for long periods, thus supposedly reducing muscular action and motor activity. Rush's theory was that restraint acted as a sedative to the blood vessels, tongue, and temper. None of his methods proved beneficial.

In London in 1758, the prominent English physician William Battie wrote his *Treatise on Madness* and founded St. Luke's Hospital for the mentally ill. Around 1793, the British merchant William Tuke and the French physician Philippe Pinel worked diligently to improve conditions and to establish treatment programs in mental institutions in their respective countries. Pinel established a care regimen to replace common treatments such as bloodletting and ducking (in which people were held under water until they were on the verge of drowning), and his work became the foundation of the modern-day humanistic theory. Despite these positive steps, by the beginning of the nineteenth century, conditions in asylums in America and in Europe generally remained deplorable, and it was only public outcries that eventually led to reform. At age 39, Dorothea Lynde Dix (1802–1887), an American woman who had been institutionalized briefly, began a huge reform movement by bringing asylum conditions to the public eye. She investigated conditions in institutions in America and Europe, and her 40-year campaign resulted in the construction of more than thirty hospitals for the indigent mentally ill (Figure 1.2).

Foundations of Neuropathology and Psychology   By the early 1800s, modern psychology had begun to develop, and it progressed during the century from a predominantly philosophical study of mental illness to a scientific

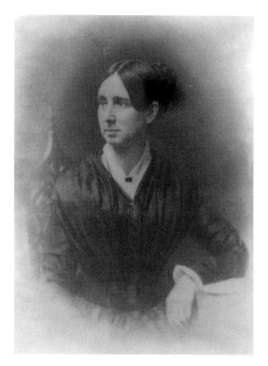

Figure 1.2
Dorothea Lynde Dix (1802–1887): "There are few cases in history where a social movement of such proportions can be attributed to the work of a single individual." (Murphy and Kovach, 1972. Courtesy Library of Congress Prints and Photographs Division.)

study. In Germany, Wilhelm Wundt (1832–1930), commonly credited as the founder of scientific psychology, created the first teaching and research laboratory. The ancient Greek and Roman tradition of treating mental illness medically had again become standard practice by the late 1800s, and a clear distinction began to form between psychoses and neuroses. German psychiatrist Emil Kraepelin (1856–1926), a student of Wundt, followed his instructor's lead and studied neurological changes in the brain. He developed a method for grouping mental illness by both causes and symptoms and differentiated between manic-depressive psychosis, dementia, and dementia praecox (later called schizophrenia). His classification system became the basis of the DSM. One of Kraepelin's colleagues, Alois Alzheimer (1864–1915), identified the plaques and tangles in the brain by which Alzheimer's disease, one form of dementia and a mental illness, is definitively identified through autopsy. These men became legendary figures in the field now known as the neurosciences (although the word had then not yet been created).

Meanwhile, two psychologists Pierre Janet (1859–1949) and Sigmund Freud (1856–1939)—often considered two of the most influential in the field—were developing theories about another group of disorders: neuroses. Janet believed neurotic people had insufficient mental energy to maintain integration of their psyches and, therefore, some parts of the psyche acted in disassociation from other parts. Freud theorized that strong, diverse, and conflicting unconscious forces influenced behavior and personality. He developed talk therapy and free association, in which his patients spoke freely of whatever came to mind. Although they were—and still are—highly controversial and often rejected, his philosophies and methods became the basis for the modern psychoanalytic theory.

Twentieth Century and Beyond

The twentieth century brought major developments in psychiatry and psychotherapy, surgical interventions, pharmaceuticals, brain imaging, and research into genetic and environmental influences, all in the ongoing attempt to better understand, diagnose, and treat—and perhaps prevent—mental illness. These subjects are discussed further in Chapters 3 and 4.

PREVALENCE IN MODERN SOCIETY

The incidence of mental illness throughout the world has been greatly underestimated, as has its emotional and financial burden.

Global Burden of Disease

An unprecedented survey by Harvard University and the World Health Organization (WHO) commissioned by the World Bank in the early 1990s resulted in a report titled "Global Burden of Disease," summarized in a book of the same name published in 1996. The survey calculated the burden of disease—the social and economic costs of particular medical conditions—in disability-adjusted life years (DALYs), defined in Table 1.1. It found that in 1990, mental illness, including suicide, created 15 percent of the total burden of disease in the United States and other developed countries, ranking second only to cardiovascular disease.

Four mental disorders—bipolar disorder, major depression, obsessive-compulsive disorder, and schizophrenia—are among the ten leading causes of disability. In Australia in 1997, mental disorders, including drug dependency, incurred the greatest burden of disease, affecting 27 percent of individuals between the ages of 18 and 24. The National Institute of Mental Health (NIMH) estimates that in the U.S. popula-

Table 1.1   Disease Burden by Selected Illness Categories in Established Market Economies, 1990

	Percent of Total DALYs*
All cardiovascular conditions	18.6
All mental illness	15.4
All malignant diseases (cancer)	15.0
All respiratory conditions	4.8
All alcohol use	4.7<
All infectious and parasitic diseases	2.8
All drug use	1.5

*Disability-adjusted life year (DALY) is a measure that expresses years of life lost to premature death and years lived with a disability of specified severity and duration (Murray & Lopez, 1996).

tion in any particular year, mental illness affects 22.1 percent of people 18 years of age and older (one in five adults). In 1998, that equaled approximately 44.3 million adults. The WHO's "World Health Report 2001" predicted that one in every four people worldwide will suffer some form of mental illness during his or her lifetime, with higher-income countries experiencing a higher rate than low-income countries (Figure 1.3).

In the United States, the most serious mental disorders, primarily major depressive disorders, which can occur simultaneously with anxiety disorders and substance abuse, affect approximately 5 percent of adults (almost 10 million) and 9 percent of children (approximately 5 million) in any given year. Women are twice as likely as men to suffer depressive disorders, at averages of 12 percent and 6.6 percent of the population, respectively. A 2005 survey by Harvard Medical School indicated that approximately half the adult population in the United States will at some point in their lives meet the DSM-IV criteria for a mental disorder. The report states that the most serious disorders manifest by the age of 14, and three-fourths of adults who develop mental illnesses will do so by the age of 24. NAMI predicts that major depressive illnesses will be the greatest cause of disability among women and children worldwide by 2020.

Costs

The enormous cost of mental illness to society is virtually beyond calculation. It creates a crushing financial burden to sufferers and their families, not to mention the emotional costs, which are also enormous and cannot be assessed monetarily. It also has huge financial ramifications on

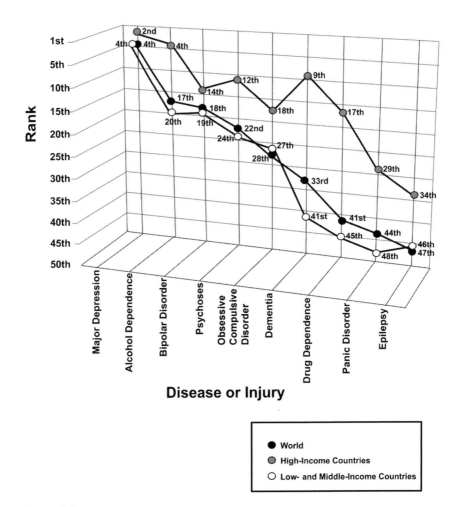

Figure 1.3
Rank of selected mental disorders among all causes of disease burden: estimates for 1998. (Ricochet Productions, after *The World Health Report* 1999, Annex Table 3.)

the nation's economy in both direct and indirect costs. The highest percentage of costs related to mental illness in the United States is attributable to two of the most severe forms: schizophrenia, which affects approximately 2.2 million people, and bipolar disorder (manic-depressive illness), which affects approximately 2.3 million. The surgeon general's report on mental health, published in 1999, found that the majority of those who need it will not seek treatment. One reason is that treatment is expensive. However, while the cost of treatment (a direct cost) may be high, the cost of nontreatment (an indirect cost) is much higher.

Direct Costs   The United States spent $49 billion for direct treatment of mental illnesses in 1991. That grew to $69 billion in 1996, of which public payers (governments and government-funded organizations) spent approximately $37 billion (53 percent). Private sources spent $32 billion (47 percent), $18 billion of which came from private insurance companies. The remainder was out-of-pocket payments, such as insurance copayments by individuals, prescriptions not covered by Medicare, and direct payments by uninsured individuals or those choosing not to use their medical coverage (Figure 1.4).

By 2001, direct costs in the United States associated with mental illness had reached $85 billion. Mental health expenditures as a portion of total health care expenditures rose by 6.7 percent, compared with 6.4 percent for all health care, between 1996 and 2001 (Figure 1.5). Several factors appear to be driving the growth in mental health costs: more people are seeking treatment; prices for psychotropic medications and the number of people using them have increased; and the unit cost of mental health services, such as hourly wages for employees in substance-abuse centers and psychiatric hospitals, has increased.

Indirect Costs   Of the approximately 450 million people worldwide who suffer from some form of mental or neurological disorder, approximately two-thirds of those who are actually aware they are ill are not receiving treat-

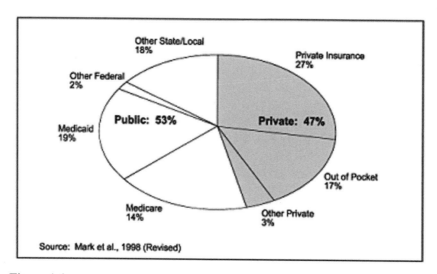

Figure 1.4
Mental health expenditures by payer, 1996 (total: $69 billion). (Ricochet Productions.)

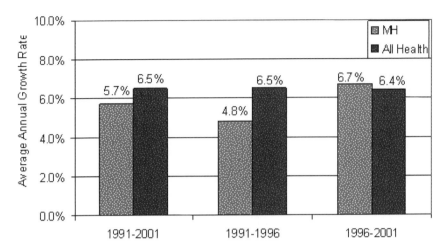

Figure 1.5
Growth in mental health (MH) expenditures compared with all health expenditures from 1991 through 2001 and in 5-year increments. (Ricochet Productions, after National Expenditures for Mental Health Services and Substance Abuse Treatment, 1991–2001.)

ment. Indirect costs related to mental illness, which include homelessness, unemployment, inability to continue working, decreased productivity, crime, incarceration, welfare programs, and suicide, are primarily due to lack of treatment. The surgeon general's report on mental health conservatively estimated the level of these indirect costs in the United States in 1990 at almost $79 billion (according to the most recent records then available). In the United States, the suicide rate rises from 1 percent in the general population to 15–17 percent in individuals with psychotic or extreme depressive disorders. Costs due to premature death were approximately $12 billion; to lost productivity among the living mentally ill, approximately $63 billion; and to incarceration or individuals caring for a family member, approximately $4 billion.

Approximately 300,000 incarcerated individuals (16 percent) suffer from serious, untreated brain disorders and psychotic thinking, many of whom have committed serious crimes, including homicides, although the majority have committed more minor offenses. They are incarcerated twice as long and are more likely to commit suicide than are inmates without mental illnesses. In 1996, the Department of Justice estimated that the cost of incarceration of the mentally ill—not including court, ambulance, emergency room, law enforcement, or social services expenses—had grown to $15 billion.

Of the estimated 600,000 homeless in the United States, 200,000 (33 percent) have untreated psychiatric disturbances, which are obviously a major cause of homelessness. Those with psychotic illnesses are frequent victims of crimes, including violent crimes such as rape and murder. Such crimes most often are not reported or, when they are, receive little attention from officials, and the resultant personal suffering is a cost that cannot be calculated.

ABUSES OF PSYCHIATRY AND OF THE MENTALLY ILL

Historically, people with mental illnesses were mistreated, stigmatized, and neglected, and, in many cases, they still are.

Involuntary Commitment

One highly controversial issue surrounding mental illness is involuntary commitment, a legal practice that allows persons to be placed in a psychiatric institution or ward without their informed consent or against their will. All states in the United States and many countries throughout the world have enacted laws governing this practice. In most instances, involuntary commitment is reserved for individuals who require treatment but whose illness affects their reasoning abilities so greatly that the decision for institutionalized treatment is made for them within a specified legal framework. Some frameworks allow involuntary commitment only if the individual is deemed a serious risk either to themselves (e.g., having suicidal thoughts) or to society (e.g., displaying homicidal tendencies), and the individual must be assessed by a psychiatrist. Even so, opponents to involuntary commitment argue against it on the grounds that the practice can be, and is, used as a means to rid society of undesirable individuals. This can occur in individual situations and involve personal motives, or it can be used on a widespread basis as a political tool.

Political Abuse of Psychiatry

In the late 1800s, German authorities were already ordering compulsory sterilization of people with mental handicaps. Adolph Hitler encouraged passage of a law in 1933 expanding the practice to other segments of society as part of his efforts to cleanse Germany of those he personally considered unfit to live or to produce offspring. The mentally ill, and many others who were arbitrarily declared to be mentally ill by psychiatrists who either supported Hitler's goal or were coerced to do so, were committed to psychiatric institutions through an involuntary commitment program. Hitler developed the T4 euthanasia program in 1939, in which psychiatrists at all psychiatric hospitals were ordered to identify those

patients with mental and hereditary disorders, those who had been hospitalized for more than 5 years, those of Jewish origin, and those meeting
certain other criteria. The selected patients were bused to special hospitals
equipped with gas chambers and were exterminated. The T4 euthanasia
program was the genesis of the Holocaust.

In the late 1970s and early 1980s, the world became aware that the
Soviet Union, Romania, and some other eastern European countries were
politically misusing psychiatry to oppress and silence dissenters and religious followers by labeling them mentally ill and committing them to
psychiatric institutions against their will. In the late 1990s, the World
Psychiatric Association (WPA); the U.S. Department of State's Bureau of
Democracy, Human Rights and Labor; and other international agencies
turned their attention on similar serious abuses in China.

Efforts by international organizations, national governments, nongovernmental organizations (NGOs), and advocacy groups to stop the
political abuse of psychiatry are ongoing. In 1974, the first international
committee was formed to this end; it eventually became the Geneva Initiative on Psychiatry (GIP). The WPA officially condemned political misuse
of psychiatry in 1977 and established ethical standards by which psychiatrists worldwide must practice.

In 2002, the World Medical Association (WMA) became concerned for
political dissidents in several countries who were detained in psychiatric
institutions and undergoing unnecessary psychiatric treatment as punishment. The WMA declared such detention and treatment unacceptable. It
called for psychiatrists and physicians in these countries, many of whom
are coerced by their governments, to resist involvement in such abusive
practices; for member medical associations to help physicians resist; for
governments to stop the abuse of using psychiatry and medicine for political
objectives; and for NGOs and the WHO to support its resolution.

Human Rights for the Mentally Ill

The Network of Reformers in Psychiatry was established 1993 to
address mental health care reform in central and eastern Europe and to
coordinate more than 600 mental health care reformers in twenty-nine
countries. Despite this effort, many mentally ill people in the region and
throughout the world continue to suffer under inhumane conditions. In
some Russian cities, mentally ill prisoners are kept in conditions reminiscent of the Middle Ages and, due to the lack of staff and medication, remain
untreated. In India, the National Human Rights Commission (NHRC)
found that in 38 percent of India's psychiatric hospitals, patients lived in
jail-like conditions, and less than 50 percent of those hospitals had any type

of mental health care professional on staff; in 2001, twenty-eight patients in one hospital died in a fire while chained to pillars. Similar conditions exist in many other countries: in 1996, the Italian government ordered ninety-seven mental asylums closed due to horrific conditions and patient neglect; in 1999, intolerable conditions in Mexican asylums were exposed. Mental Disability Rights International (MDRI), based in Washington, D.C., has documented human rights abuses against the mentally ill in twenty-three countries, including Peru, Kosovo, Hungary, Uruguay, and Paraguay.

Governmental and private organizations and advocate groups around the world work diligently to protect the human rights of the mentally ill. In June 2005, WHO—which estimates that up to 25 percent of countries worldwide either have no mental health legislation or do not enforce it if they do—published the *WHO Resource Book on Mental Health, Human Rights and Legislation*, which sets forth standards of legislation and urges all countries to pass protection laws for the mentally ill. The organization also offers professional advice and technical services to support its efforts. WHO's director general, Lee Jong-Wook, commented: "We have a moral and legal obligation to modernize mental health legislation."

Abuses in the United States

In the United States, between 1907 and 1939, in what appears reminiscent of historical events in Germany, more than 30,000 people in mental institutions or prisons were sterilized, most against their will or without their knowledge. In New Orleans, in the 1950s, psychiatrist Robert Heath of Tulane University and Australian psychiatrist Harry Bailey performed barbaric psychosurgical experiments on African American prisoners by implanting electrodes into their brains. Heath, funded by the Central Intelligence Agency (CIA), also experimented in the name of psychiatry with the potent drugs LSD and bulbocapnine, which he used on African American prisoners at the Louisiana State Penitentiary without their knowledge. Many were so severely traumatized that they never fully recovered. Also in the 1950s at the National Institutes of Mental Health Addiction Research Center in Kentucky, experiments with LSD were performed on African American drug addicts. At this same center in the 1960s, BZ, an experimental drug that was 100 times stronger than LSD, was tested on healthy African American men. A statement by the international watchdog organization Citizens Commission on Human Rights (CCHR) states, "This follows a long psychiatric tradition of using for experimental purposes the incarcerated, the dispossessed and others who have no voice."

In 1997, mentally ill inmates in the Iowa state penitentiary lived under such horrific conditions that a U.S. district judge ordered reforms, and although a 200-bed clinical care unit was built in 2002, four inmate patients committed suicide between 2003 and 2004. Not until a subsequent critical report was issued by Thomas White, consulting psychologist for the National Institute of Corrections, were further reforms implemented.

Even in some of the very institutions that are supposed to treat and help them, mentally ill patients can suffer serious abuses. Disruptive or unwanted behavior is often controlled by forced administration of drugs, physical restraints, and seclusion or isolation. Although it is virtually impossible to estimate how many deaths occur due to restraint techniques, a New York survey published in 1986 reported that treatment professionals in that city ordered 2,150 instances of restraint or seclusion involving 804 patients and that between 1979 and 1982, thirty patients died from such treatment. An article published in the *American Journal of Forensic Medical Pathology* in 2000 describes two restraint-related deaths and cites a report that estimates 50–150 deaths occur every year in U.S. mental health institutions as a result of physical restraint.

The National Association for Rights Protection and Advocacy (NARPA) is an independent organization, whose primary goal is to abolish all forms of forced treatment and to empower people labeled as mentally disabled to exercise their own rights. On its Web site, the organization states the following: "Every day, behind closed doors, human rights violations are occurring on a regular basis—and Americans don't know about it. America's mental health system is still the shame of the nation."

MOVING FORWARD

Mistreatment, stigma, misunderstanding, and lack of concern too often surround mental illness and those who suffer from it. These issues need to be addressed as urgently as those of finding causes, improving treatment modalities, and searching for possible preventive measures for mental illnesses. Growing public awareness worldwide, governmental action, private organizations that provide advocacy, the exposure of inhumane treatment and the passage of legislation to punish—and, hopefully, prevent—it, and the ready availability of educational materials in many forms are all positive developments in addressing the difficult and complex issues surrounding mental illness.

CHAPTER 2

Mental Illnesses: Diagnosis and Description

There are no clinical tests to definitively diagnose mental illness. Diagnosis is determined by a clinician who asks a patient for a history and listens to a description of the patient's feelings and how those feelings affect thoughts, actions, relationships, and life overall. To help clinicians diagnose a mental illness as accurately as possible and to assist researchers and scientists in their pursuit of knowledge regarding etiology (cause) and treatment, a uniform, well-organized, readily accessible classification system is essential.

DEVELOPMENT OF DIAGNOSTIC CRITERIA

The ancient Greeks appear to have been the first to attempt formal classification of mental illnesses. Expanding Hippocrates' theory, developed in the fourth century BC, that imbalance between the four bodily humors—blood, phlegm, and yellow and black bile—caused mental disturbances, Galen (129–216 AD) grouped personality types into four different categories: choleric (hotheaded; quick to anger), melancholic (sad; depressive), phlegmatic (undemonstrative; showing little emotion), and sanguine (cheerful; optimistic). Those early theories are strikingly similar to modern psychobiological theories linking mental illness to chemical imbalances in the brain. Although many attempts were made over the ensuing centuries to classify mental illness, the birth of psychiatry as a discipline in the eighteenth century brought about a proliferation of activity. The 1840 United States census recorded only one category of mental illness: idiocy/insanity. By the time of the 1880 census, seven different categories of insanity were recognized, including melancholia, mania, and dementia.

As the field of psychiatry evolved and the understanding of mental disorders grew, it became obvious that guidelines were necessary to differentiate between normal emotions, such as transient depression and sadness, and mental disorders, such as recurring or severe depression. The need to differentiate between types of mental disorders also became obvious. German psychiatrist Emil Kraepelin, who was perhaps the most influential figure in the classification of psychiatric disorders, developed a clinical system that grouped mental illnesses by the *pattern* of symptoms rather than simply by *similarities between* symptoms. In 1917, the American Medico-Psychological Association, which was soon renamed the American Psychiatric Association (APA), collaborated with the U.S. Bureau of the Census to collect statistics from hospitals on mental disorders and developed a classification system that was based on that of Kraepelin.

The system was later expanded by the American Medical Association (AMA), which created the *Standard Classified Nomenclature of Disease.*

German psychiatrist Emil Kraepelin (1856–1926) developed a system for classifying certain mental illnesses, laying the foundation for the classification system still used in the early twenty-first century by both the DSM and the ICD. Kraepelin trained under the prominent psychologist Wilhelm Wundt, and rose quickly to become director of an eighty-bed clinic at the University of Tartu in Dorpat (now Estonia), where he studied and recorded clinical details of mentally ill patients. His long-term research led to the discovery of and differentiation between dementia praecox and manic depression. He observed that symptoms of either illness could appear in the other illness, but observed that each illness had a different pattern and course. His observations led him to believe that during the course of dementia praecox, a patient's mental function steadily—albeit erratically—declined, which was not the case in manic depression. This led to the name dementia praecox—*dementia* meaning irreversible mental decline, *praecox* meaning before its time; the subsequent realization that the disorder did not necessarily cause mental decline led to it being renamed schizophrenia. Because the two disorders could exhibit virtually the same symptoms and yet display different courses and outcomes, Kraepelin realized that grouping mental illnesses simply by types of symptoms was completely inadequate. This led him to create a classification system based on common patterns of symptoms. Kraepelin also strongly believed that mental illnesses were primarily caused by genetic and biological disorders, and he vehemently opposed Sigmund Freud's postulation that they were due to psychological issues. Kraepelin's theories were largely overshadowed by Freudian theories during the twentieth century, particularly in the United States, but as the century drew to a close, scientific research showed that biological and genetic factors are undoubtedly significant in the development of mental illnesses. Although Kraepelin's enormous contribution remains largely unacknowledged, his work carries such significance that several eminent psychologists and psychiatrists call him the founder of modern scientific psychiatry, psychiatric genetics, and psychopharmacology.

World War II brought a dramatic increase in mental illness among military personnel, and, finding the APA's classification system too restrictive, the U.S. Armed Forces expanded the diagnostic criteria. This new system was further expanded by the Veterans Administration, and by the end of the war, four competing classification systems were in use in the United States. To further complicate matters, in 1948, the World Health Organization (WHO) included its own criteria in the sixth edition of its International Classification of Diseases (ICD-6)—the first edition was published in 1900 listing ten categories for psychoses, nine for psychoneuroses, and seven for personality disorders.

Development of the *Diagnostic and Statistical Manual of Mental Disorders*

By that time, the confusion surrounding diagnostic criteria was so great that the APA, using the Armed Forces classification system as its base, began work on the *Diagnostic and Statistical Manual of Mental Disorders* (DSM) in order to develop a common system of categorization. In collaboration with the National Institute of Mental Health (NIMH), questionnaires were sent to 10 percent of the APA membership, and the nomenclature committee established categories based on symptoms. The first DSM was published in 1952. This brief manual contained 106 diagnostic categories. Each disorder was accompanied by a list of symptoms and a brief discussion on possible causes. There was no attempt to suggest types of treatment. Further developments in the field of psychiatry necessitated a revision of the original DSM, which is now referred to as the DSM-I. The revised version, the DSM-II, published in 1968 and ninety-two pages long, added seventy-six diagnostic categories, for a total of 173. Both versions were based almost entirely on the psychodynamic or psychoanalytic framework that originated primarily with Sigmund Freud (1856–1939) and evolved through the work of other prominent psychiatrists, such as Carl Jung (1875–1961), Alfred Alder (1870–1937), and Melanie Klein (1882–1960). Although each developed different approaches to psychiatry, their methods of analysis and classification were based on investigation of the interrelationship between mind and personality. The psychoanalytic approach distinguishes between neuroses and psychoses: neuroses, into which depressive and anxiety disorders are categorized, cause distortion of reality; psychoses, common in schizophrenia, cause a complete break with reality and are so severe that people suffering from them are typically unable to care for themselves. Psychotic traits include irrational and distorted thinking (delusions), seeing things that do not exist (hallucinations), and extreme concern about one's own well-being or safety (paranoia).

At this stage of the development of psychoanalytic theory, no sharp difference was drawn between normal and abnormal. Everyone was deemed to be abnormal in one way or another; how abnormal was determined by how severely the individual's ability to function was affected. Also, even though the DSM-II had an expanded diagnostic base over its predecessor, once again no treatment recommendations were included.

By the late 1960s and early 1970s, psychiatry was experiencing scathing attacks from several groups, including the antipsychiatry movement, the behaviorists, and many medical professionals, the latter adhering strongly to a physiological (organic or biological) rather than a psychological account of mental illness. Also, research brought dynamic changes to the field of psychiatry. The APA therefore set up a task force in 1974 to develop yet another revamped version of the DSM that would attempt to address such aspects as etiology, severity of symptoms, possible treatment options, and outcomes. In many ways, the DSM-III, published in 1980, was revolutionary. An innovative manual, it virtually abandoned the psychoanalytic model and adopted the biomedical model. Its 482 pages contained 256 different diagnoses and utilized, for the first time, scientific and empirical evidence (evidence based on observation, experiments, and experience), as well as information gained through the development and use of psychotherapeutic drugs. It provided clear, descriptive, diagnostic criteria organized under a multiaxial system, presented structured interviews to be used with patients, and attempted to remain neutral in the conflicts and debate surrounding etiologies. The multiaxial system, composed of five scales, took into consideration several aspects of a person's life, including family, environmental, and social aspects:

- Axis I: Clinical disorders and conditions that require clinical attention
- Axis II: Personality disorders and mental retardation
- Axis III: General medical conditions
- Axis IV: Psychosocial and environmental problems (stressors)
- Axis V: Global assessment of functioning

The DSM-III was so well accepted that revenues led to the foundation of the American Psychiatric Press. The DSM-III was revised in 1987 due to differences with the ICD in coding systems and new insights gained by research. In the DSM-III-Revised (DSM-III-R), some categories were deleted and others added, for a total of 297 different diagnoses. However, the revision created discrepancies with the DSM-III, and controversial diagnoses, such as masochistic personality disorder, paraphilic rapism, and even premenstrual syndrome, were considered too socially sensitive to be included. Again, both versions were heavily criticized by certain segments of the medical and psychiatric profession.

Due, again, to continuing advances in research and psychiatry that allowed for a more detailed and refined description and understanding of different mental disorders, the DSM-III-R was replaced by the DSM-IV in 1994. Compiling the DSM-IV was a major undertaking that drew from decades of research and input from thousands of experts from across the United States involved in every specialty and subspecialty of psychiatry. The 5-year project involved more than 1,000 researchers and clinicians nationally and internationally and was overseen by a twenty-seven-member task force of experts mandated to ensure that all diagnoses were meaningful and replicable. The task force developed thirteen work groups. Each group contained between five and fifteen members, had an advisory committee of fifty to one hundred members, and had responsibility for a section of the manual. In a three-step process, the groups conducted extensive reviews of professional literature surrounding each diagnosis, collected and analyzed data to determine the need for changes in diagnostic criteria, and conducted field trials to determine whether clinical research was pertinent to clinical practice. The field trials involved more than 7,000 patients in eighty-eight locations nationally and internationally.

The resulting publication consists of 886 pages, with 365 diagnostic categories and subcategories organized under the multiaxial system. Disorders are grouped according to similarity of symptoms, with a list of possible associated symptoms and their duration (inclusion criteria) and a list of symptoms that must not be present (exclusion criteria) given for each disorder. Each disorder is accompanied by a descriptive text organized under the following headings:

- Diagnostic features
- Subtypes and/or specifiers
- Recording procedures
- Associated features and disorders
- Specific culture, age, and gender features
- Prevalence
- Course
- Familial pattern
- Differential diagnosis

Using these diagnostic criteria increases diagnostic reliability—the likelihood that different practitioners will reach the same diagnostic conclusion. A specific numeric code is given for each disorder, which facilitates researchers and scientists in performing data collection and retrieval that is used to compile statistical studies. The codes are also used by service providers to request payment from insurance companies. The contents of the manual are accessible through classification based on diagnostic criteria as well as through a numeric code listing. The DSM-IV places greater emphasis than the DSM-III on the role of culture, age, gender, ethnicity, and environmental factors in the development, diagnosis, and assessment of mental disorders. A special section describes how symptoms may manifest differently in people from different cultures and ethnic groups and how people from different groups and cultures may describe symptoms differently. Also addressed are how substance abuse and general physical conditions influence mental illnesses. The main text is followed by eleven appendixes. Appendix A contains "decision trees," in which sets of questions help clinicians to more objectively determine the presence or absence of symptoms when forming a diagnosis. The DSM-IV is accompanied by a four-volume Sourcebook, which—among other things—carefully documents the rationale behind the manual and its criteria sets, supporting that rationale with empirical evidence.

In 2000, the APA revamped the DSM-IV and released the Text Revision (DSM-IV-TR). A relatively minor revision compared with the development of its predecessor, its changes consist primarily of new descriptions that accompany each disorder, of minor changes in the criteria sets and disorder definitions, and of changes in the diagnostic codes to keep them compatible with the ICD. Important changes from the DSM-IV are listed in Appendix D of the DSM-IV-TR. Translated into twenty-two languages, it is the most widely used psychiatric reference system in the world, and dozens of separate publications facilitate understanding and use of the manual. These publications include classification sheets, user guides, study guides, a clinicians' version, an administration version, a case book, case studies, information about differential diagnosis, quick desk references, structured clinical interviews specific to each axis, and many more. As of 2006, a new revision, the DSM-V, is scheduled for publication in 2010.

As already described, the DSM-IV-TR is an encyclopedic volume. It describes 365 different diagnostic criteria, but the continuing increase in the number of different diagnoses does not imply an increase in the basic types of mental illnesses or that greater numbers of people are being diagnosed with mental illness. It does mean, however, that the major increase in interest in and research on mental illness is allowing more precise descriptions and diagnoses and more precise distinctions between and within mental disorders to be made. In turn, more precise identification improves treatment effectiveness and aids further scientific research.

Whereas the DSM remains the most popular and widely accepted diagnostic manual, the official international classification system for both mental and physical diseases is the ICD, which also undergoes periodic revision. The ICD-10, published in 1993, is a two-volume set, with a blue book presenting clinical descriptions and a green book defining criteria. Although formatted in a manner similar to the DSM, it does not incorporate a multiaxial system. A massive revision underway as of 2006, to be titled ICD-10-Procedure Coding System (ICD-10-PCS), will incorporate the multiaxial system.

DSM Multiaxial System The DSM-IV-TR is a lengthy diagnostic manual, often considered cumbersome. To help facilitate accessibility to its information and therefore assist diagnosis, mental disorders are grouped into five major categories, called axes. A very brief summary of each axis follows.

Axis I: Clinical Disorders; Other Conditions That May Be a Focus of Clinical Attention Categories in this axis are:

1. *Disorders Usually First Diagnosed in Infancy, Childhood, or Adolescence*: includes disorders of learning, communication, motor skills, development, attention-deficit/hyperactivity, disruptive behavior, conduct, defiance, separation anxiety, and mental retardation.
2. *Delirium, Dementia, and Amnestic and Other Cognitive Disorders*: includes delirium; dementia; Alzheimer's, Parkinson's,

and Huntington's diseases; cognitive disorders; and both general medical and substance-induced amnestic disorders.

3. *Mental Disorders Due to a General Medical Condition*: includes catatonic disorders and personality changes.

4. *Substance-Related Disorders*: includes substance-use disorders (dependence and abuse); substance-induced disorders (intoxication; withdrawal; anxiety, mood, psychotic sleep, and persisting amnestic disorders; sexual dysfunction); alcohol-related disorders (abuse, dependence, intoxication delirium, persisting dementia, psychotic disorder); and numerous disorders related to amphetamines, caffeine, cannabis, cocaine, hallucinogens, inhalants, nicotine, and other substances.

5. *Schizophrenia and Other Psychotic Disorders*: includes catatonic, disorganized, paranoid, residual, and undifferentiated schizophrenia; schizoaffective, delusional, brief psychotic, and shared psychotic disorders; psychotic disorders due to a general medical condition; and substance-induced psychotic disorder.

6. *Mood Disorders*: includes major depressive disorder; manic, hypomanic, or mixed episodes; single or recurrent depressive episodes; bipolar disorders; and substance- or illness-induced mood disorders.

7. *Anxiety Disorders*: includes acute stress, generalized anxiety, obsessive-compulsive, agoraphobia without panic, panic with and without agoraphobia, and post-traumatic disorders.

8. *Somatoform Disorders*: includes conversion, pain, and somatization disorders and hypochondriasis.

9. *Factitious Disorders*: in which individuals intentionally act physically or mentally ill without receiving any obvious benefits. These disorders can be psychological, physical, a combination of both, or not otherwise specified (NOS).

10. *Dissociative Disorders*: which manifest as disruption in the functions of consciousness, memory, identity, or perception of the environment. This category includes amnesia, depersonalization, and identity.

11. *Sexual and Gender Identity Disorders*: includes disorders of sexual desire (aversion, hypoactive), arousal, orgasmic function, sexual dysfunction (substance-induced or due to general medical condition), and gender identity. It also includes paraphilias, exhibitionism, pedophilia, masochism, and sadism.

12. *Eating Disorders*: includes anorexia nervosa, bulimia nervosa, and eating disorders NOS.

13. *Sleep Disorders*: includes breathing-related, circadian rhythm, nightmare, sleep terror, and sleepwalking disorders; dyssomnia; hypersomnia; insomnia; and narcolepsy.

14. *Impulse-Control Disorders Not Elsewhere Classified*: includes klep-tomania, pathological gambling, and pyromania.
15. *Adjustment Disorders (with)*: depressed mood, anxiety, conduct dis-turbances, mixed anxiety and depressed mood, mixed disturbances of emotions and conduct, and other unspecified disorders.

Axis II: Personality Disorders   Disorders in this category are grouped as follows:

Cluster A: paranoid, schizoid, and schizotypal disorders.
Cluster B: antisocial, borderline, histrionic, and narcissistic disorders.
Cluster C: avoidant, dependent, and obsessive-compulsive disorders.
Personality Disorder not otherwise specified.
Other Conditions That May Be a Focus of Clinical Attention, including:

- Psychological factors affecting medical condition
- Medication-induced disorders
- Relational problems: related to a mental disorder or general med-ical condition; parent-child; partner; sibling
- Problems related to abuse or neglect: physical and sexual abuse of a child or adult; child neglect
- Additional conditions such as noncompliance with treatment; adult, child, or adolescent antisocial behavior; age-related cogni-tive decline; bereavement; and identity, religious or spiritual, acculturation, and phase-of-life problems.

Axis III: General Medical Conditions

Axis IV: Psychosocial and Environmental Problems

Axis V: Global Assessment of Functioning Scale

Description of Some Mental Disorders

To be diagnosed as a mental disorder, the suspected disorder must *significantly* interfere with a person's ability to function in a particular area.

Schizophrenia   Of the 365 diagnostic categories in the DSM-IV-TR, schizophrenia is the most cruel, severe, and disabling, and those suffering with it are fifty times more likely to commit suicide that those in the gen-eral population. It is a highly complex and an as yet poorly understood condition, the root causes of which continue to be debated but are virtually unknown. It is believed that a chemical imbalance in the brain plays a significant role; however, what causes this imbalance remains a mystery. Studies have shown that two factors—genetic (hereditary) and perinatal (associated with pregnancy)—may be significant in the development of schizophrenia.

- *Genetic:* There is a higher incidence of this disorder among family members. First-degree relatives (parents, siblings, offspring) of a person with schizophrenia have a 10 percent risk of developing the disorder. Children of parents who both have schizophrenia have a 40 or 50 percent risk. In dizygotic (fraternal) twins, the risk of both developing it is 10 percent—similar for that between sisters and brothers—whereas risk is as high as 40–50 percent for monozygotic (identical) twins. Schizophrenia has also been associated with being left-handed.
- *Perinatal*: A good deal of research has been conducted surrounding the association between schizophrenia and pregnancy and birth complications. It appears that some women who are malnourished or who contract certain viral illnesses, such as the flu, during pregnancy, particularly during the first trimester, may be at higher risk of having children who develop schizophrenia. For this reason, it is possible that children born during the winter may be at higher risk. Complications during pregnancy may also be a risk factor. These factors suggest schizophrenia is a neurodevelopmental disorder; however, again, the processes are poorly understood.

Schizophrenia is a chronic brain disease that affects 3.4 of every 1,000 people in the United States annually—more than 2 million in any single year—with 100,000 new cases diagnosed every year. As seen in Chapter 1, it is one of four mental disorders that combined make up the top ten causes of disability from all medical conditions in developed countries. Schizophrenia is prevalent worldwide although rates are lower in south European countries and in most developing nations. It affects women and men with equal frequency although men tend to develop it earlier (by their late teens or early twenties) than women do (usually in their twenties to early thirties). Although children over the age of 5 years can develop schizophrenia, it is very rare among children. The disorder seems to have no racial preference. Symptoms usually develop gradually although onset can also be sudden, and family and friends usually notice symptoms before the individual does. Although environmental (social) stressors seem to intensify symptoms, they do not cause the disorder.

Symptoms of schizophrenia ebb and flow and are divided into three basic phases: prepsychotic, psychotic, and postpsychotic. In all phases, the core problem is social and/or occupational impairment. Another is apathy. In both the pre- and postpsychotic phases, patients experience a plethora of associated symptoms, which can include the following:

- Appetite or eating problems
- Depressed or sad mood
- Fatigue
- Feelings of guilt or worthlessness
- Hyperactivity
- Hostility
- Impulsive or reckless behavior
- Obsessive/compulsive thoughts and behavior
- Poor attention or concentration abilities
- Prolonged anxiety

When severe, these symptoms can lead to serious consequences that affect an individual's life, among which are unemployment, money management difficulties, poor hygiene and grooming, self-injury, impaired learning and memory, and institutionalization. In fact, estimates suggest that hospitalization for schizophrenia accounts for approximately 30 percent of all hospital beds—not just those in psychiatric hospitals—in the United States.

The psychotic phase is accompanied by terrifying symptoms and devastating impairments, distorting thought and perception so severely that the individual virtually loses contact with reality. These symptoms are called *psychoses*, which are characterized primarily by hallucinations, delusions, paranoia, and disorganized thought patterns that manifest in bizarre behavior and speech, and often by decreased movement, speech, and emotions.

Hallucinations are things seen, heard, felt, smelled, or tasted that are not actually there but are perceived as being absolutely real. When experiencing auditory hallucinations, for example, people with schizophrenia often—sometimes continually—hear voices that are not there. The voices often appear to come from somewhere outside, not from inside, the person's head. Voices can be perceived as conversations among other people or as insults, compliments, or orders directed at the individual. Some individuals describe voices as a tape playing in their head. Others believe someone has implanted some kind of broadcasting device in their brain. The voices may tell them that they are bad or evil, or that loved ones are doing bad things; or the voices may be grandiose, telling the individuals they are Jesus or some other famous person.

Delusions consist of false, internal beliefs that are based on an incorrect perception or misinterpretation of the real, external environment; they are beliefs held by that particular individual and no one else. Such beliefs are firmly held regardless of evidence or proof to the contrary. For example, a schizophrenic person may believe that being bumped accidentally in a crowd is part of a deliberate government plot to persecute him or her. Trying to convince the person that the delusion is just that will only cause more anger and mistrust, particularly toward the person trying to do the convincing.

Disorganized thought patterns, which produce disorganized speech and behavior, can be so disjointed that the individual becomes virtually incomprehensible. Sentences become disconnected, the story being told has no point or relevance to the conversation or topic at hand, and whole words are often perceived as separate sounds, and in turn, the perceived separate sounds are perceived as separate (therefore additional) words, causing the individual to switch topics in mid-conversation. This is also known as "flight of ideas" or "derailment."

Psychotic symptoms may be preceded, accompanied, or followed by less obvious symptoms, such withdrawal, isolation, or unusual thinking and speech. Some patients experience only one psychotic episode. Most, however, are chronic sufferers and experience many psychotic episodes over their lifetime. These episodes are called *relapses* or *acute periods*. During an acute period or relapse, psychotic sensations, such as hallucinations, delusions, and confused thought, occur in addition to the usual disruptive thoughts and feelings and are thus called *positive symptoms* (which are by no means "positive" in the sense of being good). Acute periods are followed by periods of remission during which a patient may lead a relatively normal life. However, these periods of convalescence are often accompanied by a reduction of normal feelings—loss of interest, affection, humor, and energy—which are thus called *negative symptoms*. Typically, the chronic sufferer does not regain normal functioning, and long-term treatment—with medication thought to be the most effective—is necessary to control symptoms. The 30-year treatment success rate is as follows:

- 25 percent completely recover
- 35 percent are much improved and able to live relatively independently
- 15 percent are improved but require an extensive support network
- 10 percent are unimproved and are hospitalized
- 15 percent are dead, primarily from suicide

Because symptoms can vary, several subcategories of schizophrenia have been developed. One is *paranoid schizophrenia*, in which psychotic episodes are accompanied by *paranoia*, a strong feeling that one is being watched, followed, or persecuted and that others speak badly of or wish to harm one. *Disorganized schizophrenia* manifests as verbal incoherence, with emotions and moods that are highly inappropriate for the situation in which they occur; hallucinations and delusions are not usually present in this type of schizophrenia. *Catatonic schizophrenia* is marked by extreme withdrawal, negativity, and self-isolation. The diagnosis of catatonic requires that the patient display disrupted psychomotor activity (muscle movements directly proceeding from mental activities) as a dominant feature. These psychomotor disturbances may swing between extremes, such as abnormally increased and virtually uncontrollable muscular movements (hyperkinesis), and a trance-like state of unconsciousness; or they may manifest as a type of automatic obedience. These states may be present for long periods, and episodes of violent excitement may occur. Individuals diagnosed with *undifferentiated schizophrenia* meet the general criteria for schizophrenia while not meeting the requirements for the other specific subtypes. Individuals diagnosed with this subtype usually express no motivation, initiative, emotional responsiveness, social interest, or enjoyment.

When psychotic episodes are accompanied by symptoms of other mental disorders, particularly prolonged periods of euphoria (mania) or depression, or both—which are symptoms of certain mood disorders—clinicians are presented with the difficulty of discerning whether the patient has two separate illnesses, a combination of the two, or perhaps even an illness that is distinct from both schizophrenia and mood disorder. Therefore, when features of both illnesses are present but the diagnostic criteria for neither one are completely met, the patient is usually diagnosed with *schizoaffective disorder*. This disorder is not classified as schizophrenia, and certain of its symptoms are associated with the category of personality disorders, which includes *schizoid personality, schizophreniform disorder*, and *schizotypal personality*. Bipolar disorder, a mood disorder, is frequently misdiagnosed as schizophrenia and vice versa. Also, a particular type of autism, Asperger's syndrome, is often misdiagnosed as schizophrenia. Accurate diagnosis of schizophrenia and its subtypes is imperative in order for the patient to receive essential, appropriate treatment.

Scott and Schizophrenia

After living an active, productive, and successful life for 17 years, Scott developed schizophrenia. Before being diagnosed, he attempted suicide by jumping from a bridge. Only during treatment for his serious injuries was his mental illness discovered. Here is part of his frightening experience:

You can't imagine what it's like. My whole life has changed. It is like I woke up and found myself living in hell. Almost everyone around me is like a demon who is tormenting me. . . . Everyone is making fun of me all the time. Mom and Dad wouldn't believe it if I told them how bad it really is. . . . Kevin and Clyde, my two best friends . . . have turned against me. It would be OK if they just decided not to be my friends and left me alone. But they want to torment me too . . . I don't know why. I never did anything to them. We used to have such a good time, getting together to fix up our car, listening to music, and stuff like that. Now they are sending electrical signals from the car battery. It shouldn't be that strong, for a 12-volt battery, but they can actually give me electrical shocks on my skin. I don't know how they transmit the current through the air, even through walls. But they do. Sometimes they even hit my nipples. . . . If I told anyone that this was happening, they probably wouldn't believe that it was happening, they probably wouldn't believe it. . . . I'm so confused. I am so scared. I can't describe this to anyone. I have to deal with this alone. I used to be one of the guys. But now I'm an outcast. Why is this happening? What did I do? I've completely lost control over who I am, what I do, what I think. God, I've got to do something to stop what's happening to me, but I don't even know what it is. Could it really be that I am losing my mind, like one of those people in One Flew Over the Cuckoo's Nest? *If I am, then I should just kill myself. I don't want to keep living if it is going to be this bad the rest of my life.*

Nancy C. Andreasen, *Brave New Brain*, p. 186

With love, support, and understanding from family and friends, medication, and periods of hospitalization during relapses into the psychotic stages of his illness, Scott stabilized enough to hold a part-time job and take occasional college classes. However, the illness continued to smolder under the surface, and his once sunny disposition never fully returned.

Mood Disorders   *Mood* can be described as the way a person feels emotionally—sad, happy, angry, frustrated. Although everyone experiences many different types of moods, which are themselves normal and healthy human emotions, a mood disorder can be defined as a serious deviation from the normal experience that is severe enough and that persists long enough to significantly interfere with a person's life. Four of the most prevalent mood disorders are major depressive disorder, bipolar disorder, dysthymia, and cyclothymia.

Major Depressive Disorder   The syndrome of depression has been recognized for centuries. Whereas depression can range from mild to severe, major depressive disorder—also called unipolar major depression, and often simply depression—is highly debilitating. Although it is also highly treatable, the majority of people suffering major depressive disorder never seek treatment. As seen in Chapter 1, globally, major depression causes the fourth-highest burden of disease among all medical diseases, and by 2020, it is expected to rise to second place, preceded only by cardiovascular disease. Major depressive disorder already has the second-highest burden of disease in high-income countries such as the United States. In any given year, approximately 19 million adults in the United States (10 percent) will experience depressive illness, and half of them will suffer from a major depressive disorder. Major depressive disorder has been described as a "whole-body illness" because it affects not just mood, thoughts, and feelings—particularly feelings about oneself—but also how a person feels physically. It results in marked functional impairment and disabling physical symptoms and is a leading cause of decreased productivity and absenteeism in the workforce.

Criteria for diagnosis of this disorder include depressed mood accompanied by abnormal loss of interest or enjoyment for most of the day, every day, for at least two consecutive weeks. Also, five of nine symptoms must be experienced during the same 2-week-long depressed period, which include abnormal feelings of guilt, sleep disturbance, activity disturbance, poor concentration, and fatigue. A depressive episode may begin suddenly or develop slowly and may occur just once or many times throughout a person's life.

Major depressive disorder is often described as *clinical depression*. It is distinct from normal feelings of sadness, the blues, or even short-lived depression. Sadness and the blues are only rarely and briefly accompanied by feelings of hopelessness, helplessness, or worthlessness, or by the inability to feel pleasure or a positive change in mood in relation to a positive situation—all of which are symptoms of major depression. Suicidal thoughts often accompany major depression, and suicidal tendencies or symptoms of psychotic episodes, such as hallucinations or delusions, are always signs of pathological depression.

Emotional traumas are major triggers of depression. Such traumas can include significant life changes, loss of a loved one, loss of a job, financial difficulties, and stress (even desired stress). Genetic, biological, psychological, and environmental/social stressors seem to play a role in the onset of depression as well. Major depression can also be triggered by physical conditions, such as stroke, heart attack, cancer, or medication, but depression due to these types of triggers are given a separate classification within the group of mood disorders.

Major depressive disorder appears to evolve over time. Following the first depressive episode, subsequent episodes can be triggered by much more minor life situations or even occur spontaneously with no stressor present at all. Of all people who experience one major depressive episode, 80–90 percent will experience another within the following 2 years, and 50 percent of those people will experience further recurrence. With recurrence, the depressive episodes evolve into major depression, and each recurrence increases the risk of the disorder becoming chronic, which in turn increases the risk of disability and suicide.

Suicide risk increases during depression: between 10 and 15 percent of individuals who have been hospitalized at some time due to depression eventually commit suicide, and 60 percent of all suicides occur among people suffering from major depressive disorder. The lifetime risk of suicide in individuals suffering severe depression may be as high as 6 percent, considerably higher than the 1.3 percent lifetime risk in the general population.

Comorbidity, or coexistence, of mood disorders is common. Upward of 50 percent of people suffering from major depressive disorder also experience symptoms of anxiety disorder, such as panic attacks, excessive fears about health, or phobias; approximately 33 percent experience a full-blown anxiety disorder, most often a social phobia, panic disorder, or obsessive-compulsive disorder. The combination of anxiety and major depression worsens an individual's ability to be functional, decreases treatment effectiveness, and increases the risk of suicide.

Women and Depression   In the United States, more than twice as many women (approximately 12.4 million) as men (6.4 million) experience depressive disorders, and approximately 10–15 percent of all new mothers experience postpartum depression. Studies show no distinction between sufferers based on race, ethnic background, or economic status.

In fact, ten other countries have reported similar female-to-male ratios. Women between 18 and 45 years of age make up the majority of people with a major depressive disorder, and women are particularly susceptible following childbirth. Although the reason for this ratio is unclear, researchers suspect that several factors highly specific to women may be responsible, including hormonal and other biological factors, certain psychological and personality characteristics, and subjection to abuse and oppression. However, many women experiencing these conditions do not experience depression, and therefore, genetic predisposition may also be a factor.

Men and Depression Although fewer men than women are diagnosed with major depressive disorder, men are more likely to commit suicide due to depression. Although more women attempt suicide, the rate of suicide in men is four times that in women. The suicide rate for men increases after age 70, and the highest rates in the United States occur among white men older than 85. Physicians are less likely to suspect depression in men, and men are much less likely to admit to it. Even when they do, they are less likely to seek treatment. In men, depression is often disguised by drug or alcohol abuse, and even by excessively long work hours. Feelings of hopelessness or helplessness that accompany depression are less prevalent in men than in women, often being replaced by anger, irritability, and discouragement. Although the risk of coronary heart disease is increased by depression in both women and men, men are more likely to die from it.

Elderly and Depression In the United States, approximately 6 million people aged 65 and older suffer from depression. However, because depression in the elderly is often wrongly dismissed as a normal function of aging, many depressed elderly remain undiagnosed, and an estimated 90 percent of the depressed elderly are untreated. This causes much needless suffering for individuals who otherwise could lead a fulfilling remainder of their lives. Also making diagnosis difficult, the depressed elderly seem to resist admitting to feelings of hopelessness or helplessness, to unusually long periods of grief following a loss, or to other emotional conditions that are significant in depression. They focus, instead, on physical manifestations that can occur due to age or that are perhaps due to the depression, and physicians therefore often misdiagnose a patient who would otherwise respond to simple treatment methods. Depression in older adults causes a high percentage of suicide: 19 percent of all suicides occur in individuals 65 years of age and older. Although the risk of suicide is higher in white men, the suicide rate in all individuals between the ages of 80 and 84 is twice that in the general population. Among the risk factors associated with depression in the elderly are being a woman, being unmarried (particularly being widowed), living alone, lacking a supportive social network, and chronic pain, stroke, dementia, medications, and substance abuse.

Children and Depression   Major depressive disorder, along with dysthymic disorder and bipolar disorder, is one of the most frequently diagnosed mood disorders in children. The belief that children have nothing to be depressed about is now known to be a myth, but it was not until close to the 1980s that depression in children was taken seriously. Often, children are faced with situations that they are emotionally unequipped to deal with and about which they may feel powerless or perhaps even guilty—situations such as poverty, abuse, neglect, and divorce. Such feelings can precipitate depression. Young children in particular have no labels for the negative feelings they are experiencing and may just conclude that they are unlovable or stupid. They may not even realize that such feelings are abnormal. Because depression appears to be biologically based, many children are susceptible to it, regardless of the presence or absence of stressful situations.

Although childhood depression resembles depression in adults, it manifests very differently. As with the elderly, depression in children is difficult to diagnose. Depressed children often seem to be constantly sad, to no longer enjoy usual activities, and to complain frequently of physical symptoms, such as headaches and stomach aches. They may exhibit abnormal behavior patterns, such as clinging to a parent, pretending to be sick, excessively worrying about the death of a parent, refusing to go to school, performing poorly in school, and displaying negative or irritable attitudes. They may have persistent feelings of being misunderstood, exhibit low energy or the appearance of boredom, be unable to focus or concentrate, or appear hyperactive and agitated.

Diagnosing childhood depression is difficult because behavior and attitudes vary greatly between children and during different phases of the same child's development. However, researchers now believe 5 percent of children and adolescents may experience depression, and children who suffer a loss, who have a learning disorder, or who are under stress are at higher risk. Mood disorders significantly increase the risk of suicide, and suicide attempts in children peak around mid-adolescence. The rate of prevalence of actual suicide steadily increases throughout the teen years and is the third leading cause of death during those years.

Dysthymia   Dysthymia is depression that is less severe than major depressive disorder. However, it is a long-term, chronic disorder, sometimes described as "smoldering." To be diagnosed as dysthymia, depression must be present in adults for at least 2 years and in children for at least 1 year. Because it seems to manifest at an early age, as early as childhood or adolescence, it becomes such an integral part of the person's self-concept that it affects personality development, including one's coping styles, which among dysthymics are usually passive, avoidant, and dependent. These traits often cause the individual to be labeled neurotic. While dysthymia is not disabling, it prevents the afflicted from feeling good and functioning well. Many people with dysthymia are also susceptible to episodes of major depression, during which their illness is called *double depression*. Dysthymia affects approximately 2 percent of adults in the United States in any given year, and women are diagnosed twice as often as men.

Cyclothymia   Cyclothymia is a chronic mood disorder that manifests both manic and depressive episodes that are neither intense enough nor last long enough to meet the diagnostic criteria for either major depressive disorder or bipolar disorder. Onset usually occurs during adolescence or early adulthood, and although the risk of a person diagnosed with cyclothymia developing bipolar disorder is about 33 percent (thirty-three times higher than that for the general population), the rate is believed to be too low to regard cyclothymia as the forerunner of full-blown bipolar type I disorder.

Bipolar Disorder   Bipolar disorder, a recurrent and treatable mood disorder once called manic depression, is a complex disorder that can be difficult to diagnose. It affects approximately 2.3 million Americans over the age of 18 years. The disorder typically begins in young adults and continues throughout life. It manifests in one or more episodes of mania (highs) or in alternating episodes of mania and depression (lows). Episodes in either of these two poles can last for days, weeks, or even months. The manic phase—*mania* being derived from a French word meaning "frenzied" or "crazed"—is characterized by feelings of extreme elation, euphoria, and grandiosity; exaggerated self-confidence, self-importance, and optimism; by greatly increased mental and physical energy and activity; by racing thoughts and speech that skip—often incoherently—from one idea to the next; and by impulsiveness, reckless behavior, poor judgment, and a greatly diminished need for sleep without any accompanying feeling of exhaustion. The subsequent sleep deprivation can induce catatonia or a highly confused state known as *delirious mania*. In severe cases or when left untreated, mania can trigger a psychotic state in which paranoia, hallucinations, and delusions are experienced. These symptoms make bipolar disorder difficult to distinguish from schizophrenia. Because thinking and judgment are severely affected, the manic phase can also cause serious practical problems, perhaps because of poor business or financial decisions or unrestricted spending sprees, and great embarrassment, often due to wild romantic sprees and sexual indiscretions. The depressive stage manifests all the symptoms of major depressive disorders. Swings between the poles are usually gradual but can often be fast, dramatic, and severe. Bipolar disorder is less prevalent than major depressive disorders, afflicting approximately one in every 200 individuals, but the risk of suicide for those with bipolar disorder is fifteen times higher than in the general population.

Bipolar disorder is subdivided into two types:

- **Bipolar I disorder:** defined as one or more manic or mixed episodes (in which feelings of both mania and depression are experienced almost daily for at least a week) together with one or more episodes of major depression. In its most severe form, bipolar I disorder is accompanied by extreme manic episodes.
- **Bipolar II disorder:** defined as one or more depressive episodes and at least one hypomanic episode. During hypomania, symptoms are manic but less severe than during the manic episodes experienced in bipolar I disorder. However, the hypomania must be clearly distinguishable from the person's normal, nondepressed mood. Bipolar II disorder can easily be, and frequently is, misdiagnosed as depression, unless hypomania is properly identified.

Anxiety Disorders   Anxiety disorders are more common in both adults and children than any other psychiatric disorder, affecting upward of 19 million people in the United States, at a cost of more than $42 billion a year. Sufferers are six times more likely to be hospitalized for psychiatric illnesses than the general population, and because anxiety disorders produce a plethora of physical symptoms, sufferers are likely to visit a doctor three to five times more frequently than the general population. A Swedish survey by Ringback et al., published in the *Journal of Epidemiology and Community Health* in 2005, concluded that people who reported feeling abnormally anxious and nervous had a higher incidence of attempting suicide in the subsequent 5–10 years. While anxiety disorders are highly treatable, only about one-third of sufferers receive treatment.

Anxiety syndromes were probably not identified until the late 1800s, when a doctor named Jacob Mendez DaCosta described in the *American Journal of Medical Sciences* symptoms experienced by a Civil War soldier. He called the syndrome "irritable heart," and it became known as *DaCosta's syndrome*. Due to the physical symptoms of heart palpitations and chest pain (which anxiety is now known to have the ability to trigger), the disorder was erroneously thought to be of physical origin and was described as cardiac disturbances related to psychological factors such as stress. Freud was the first to recognize anxiety as the culprit for the physical manifestations, and called the syndrome *anxiety neurosis*.

Anxiety disorders, indeed, manifest in many unpleasant physical symptoms, including the following:

- Sweating
- Trembling
- Cold, clammy hands
- Nausea, intestinal problems, and diarrhea
- Difficulty swallowing
- Difficulty breathing
- Muscle tension
- Rapidly pounding heart and palpitations
- Chest pain or tightness
- Tingling in the hands and feet
- Dizziness
- Weakness

People suffering anxiety tire easily, often have difficulty sleeping, feel edgy and jumpy, are hyperalert, and—particularly those with panic disorder—can experience subjective, unprovoked attacks of panic or terror. It appears that anxiety disorders are triggered by a complicated combination of factors, such as personality, genetics, neurochemical imbalances, and environment (stressors). Of the several categories of anxiety disorders, four are

- Generalized anxiety disorder
- Panic disorder
- Obsessive-compulsive disorder
- Post-traumatic stress disorder

Generalized Anxiety Disorder A pervasive, persistent, and often chronic feeling of being anxious is typical in generalized anxiety disorder (GAD). People with GAD continuously worry uncontrollably, excessively, and disproportionately about everyday situations, which can interfere with their ability to focus, concentrate, and function effectively. GAD can be comorbid with depressive disorders, substance abuse, and other anxiety disorders, and because many of the more severe physical manifestations experienced in some anxiety disorders—such as panic attacks or obsessions—may not be present, GAD can be difficult to diagnose.

Panic Disorder   Panic attacks are sudden, unexpected, overwhelming feelings of fear that occur for no obvious reason and are accompanied by many physical manifestations typical of anxiety, in particular, feelings of suffocation, of having a heart attack, of losing control or going crazy, and of impending doom, particularly fear of dying. Some attacks last only a few minutes; others last hours. Panic disorder is a serious condition that affects approximately one in every seventy-five people and usually first manifests during the teen years or early adulthood. Major life situations seem to be triggers of panic disorder; however, genetic predisposition increases an individual's risk. It is often comorbid with agoraphobia, an anxiety disorder in which fear of having a panic attack in a place where getting out quickly would be difficult causes the individual to avoid such places.

Obsessive-Compulsive Disorder   Obsessive-compulsive disorder (OCD) is classified as an anxiety disorder because of the anxiety that occurs when the affected individual attempts to resist an obsessive or compulsive impulse. In OCD, it seems the brain gets stuck and cannot let go of particular worries, superstitions, or fears, which become so excessive that they become obsessions. An obsession can be defined as a persistent and troubling thought that the sufferer recognizes as senseless but cannot dismiss. These obsessions result in compulsive actions, which are taken in order to be rid of the obsession. For example, an obsession about being contaminated by germs can result in compulsive rituals of hours of handwashing that may continue to the point of the skin being rubbing off. OCD has been described by sufferers as continuous mental hiccups that they cannot rid themselves of.

OCD affects approximately 3.3 million, or one in fifty, adults in the United States at any given time, but almost twice that number will experience it at some time in their lives. OCD can manifest at any time between preschool age and adulthood. Studies show that it takes an average of 17 years before sufferers seek treatment. Although it is difficult to treat and is completely curable only in some people, comprehensive treatment can provide effective, long-term symptom relief. The cause of OCD remains unknown, and children of a parent with OCD are at slightly higher risk.

Post-Traumatic Stress Disorder   Post-traumatic stress disorder (PTSD) was actually first described by DaCosta when he reported on the Civil War solider with "irritable heart" syndrome. However, PTSD was not included in the modern classification system until the 1980 DSM-III. The disorder is triggered by experiencing or witnessing life-threatening situations, such as combat or concentration camps, serious accidents, natural disasters, terrorist attacks, violent personal attacks, childhood abuse or neglect, rape, and sexual molestation. Following World Wars I and II and the Korean War, its symptoms were primarily referred to as "shell shock" or "battle fatigue." The extensive number of cases that appeared after the Vietnam War brought a great deal of attention and research to the syndrome, and it is now estimated that approximately 30 percent of all people involved in combat suffer PTSD.

Predominant symptoms are "flashbacks" and episodes of reliving or reexperiencing the trauma, either through recurrent dreams and nightmares or while awake. Sleep problems and feelings of emotional detachment, psychic numbing, emotional anesthesia, and the inability to feel enjoyment are common symptoms. PTSD often occurs in conjunction with depression, memory problems, and substance abuse, and it affects an individual's ability to function effectively in the family, socially, and at work. In the United States, approximately 5.2 million adults (3.6 percent) suffer PTSD in any given year, and an estimated 7.8 percent will experience it at some time during their lives. Lifetime occurrence is estimated to be 10 percent in women and 5 percent in men. Although there is no cure, psychotherapy and certain drugs appear to be of some help.

Dementia   Dementias, often called senility, are the result of certain types of changes in brain cells. What causes those changes is as yet unknown. Dementias are characterized by deteriorating emotional and intellectual abilities, particularly memory loss, personality changes, emotional shallowness, and free and uncontrolled mood or behavioral expression of emotions. Dementias typically manifest during the fifties through seventies, but may begin as early as the forties. They are divided into four subtypes:

1. Alzheimer's disease, accounting for 50 percent of all dementias, affects roughly 4.5 million women and men in the United States older than 65, and 50 percent of people older than 85. More than 360,000 Americans are diagnosed annually, and about 50,000 annually are reported to die from it. The fastest growing segment of the population is those older than 85, and as the Baby Boom generation ages, the number of individuals with Alzheimer's disease

Estimated Number of New AD Cases, in Thousands

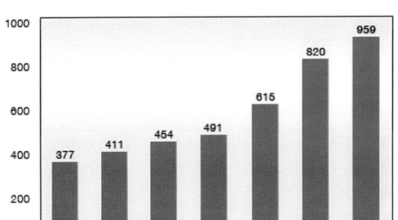

Figure 2.1
The number of Alzheimer's disease cases in the United States is expected to increase dramatically as the Baby Boom generation ages. (Ricochet Productions.)

is expected to increase drastically, to more than 14 million by 2050 (Figure 2.1).

2. Vascular conditions, including stroke or hypertension, account for about 20 percent of all dementias.
3. Substance-induced persisting dementia, the major culprit being alcohol, accounts for 7–9 percent.
4. General medical and neurological conditions account for approximately 20–30 percent. These include Huntington's chorea, which is relatively rare, and Parkinson's disease, affecting approximately 2 percent of the population.

As with other dementias, Alzheimer's is progressive and causes steady decline. Patients usually live 7–10 years, although some live for up to 15 years, after diagnosis. Unless caused by a sudden event, such as a stroke, dementias begin benignly. Although changes are at first subtle, patients notice them and become distressed. Symptoms at this stage can mimic depression, and patients are often misdiagnosed. Symptoms progress gradually over months and years, beginning with memory loss of recent events. They include impaired judgment; forgetting where personal items are; and difficulty handling money, performing simple tasks, naming objects, and understanding language. As the illness progresses, individuals get lost even when driving well-familiar roads and repeat questions frequently because the answers are forgotten almost immediately. Old memories remain at this point and become the topic of almost all conversations. Eventually they, too, fade. The patient forgets people's names, even those of spouse and children, and may undergo a drastic personality change. Responses, such as laughing or crying, become inappropriate for the situation at hand. Eventually, the patient will begin to wander off, perhaps in underwear or pajamas, and become lost. Interest in grooming and personal hygiene disappears, and ultimately the individual becomes unreachable and vegetative. The later stages are virtually a living death for the patient, and heartbreaking for loved ones. The cause of dementia is as yet not known; however, one gene has been linked to Alzheimer's risk, and high cholesterol and high blood pressure also seem to be associated with higher risk. As of 2006, there was no cure for dementia.

CHAPTER 3

Treatment Approaches to Mental Illness

Within this general, encompassing view, there can be differentiated perspectives, broader or narrower, dealing with particular aspects of man—the biological, psychodynamic, societal, and so on. These perspectives abstract certain aspects of the concrete man. They are of limited scope and usefulness, but each serves a purpose. Single perspectives do not present the complete view of man and do not tell the whole truth about him. However, they complement one another without exhausting the totality of knowledge about him and the full meaning of his existence.

Thaddeus Weckowicz, *Models of Mental Illness: Systems and Theories of Abnormal Psychology. p. 338.*

For the most part, mental illnesses are both diagnosable and treatable, with the result that most people suffering with them can live fuller, happier, more productive lives. The twentieth century yielded several distinct treatment approaches, followed by dramatic advances in those approaches and a vast array of treatment methodologies. Basically, however, methodologies can be grouped into three primary categories: psychoanalytic, behavioral, and biological.

THE PSYCHOANALYTIC APPROACH

Brief History

Perhaps the most well-known name associated with psychoanalysis in the United States—and the most controversial worldwide—is Sigmund Freud (1856–1939) (Figure 3.1). Freud was born into a Jewish family in

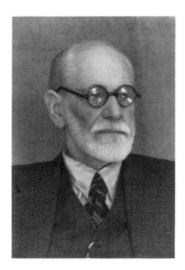

Figure 3.1
Sigmund Freud, the father of psychoanalysis. (Courtesy Library of Congress Prints and Photographs Division.)

Vienna. Once he had become a medical student, his intense desire was to enter neurophysiological research, a field in which the eminent neurologists Carl Wernicke (1848–1905), Paul Broca (1824–1880), and others were making discoveries that certain areas of the brain control certain functions. However, Freud's desire to engage in this new and exciting research was thwarted by anti-Semitism and his lack of independent wealth. He therefore trained to enter private practice, specializing in neurology.

While in training, Freud became friends with fellow physician and physiologist Josef Breuer (1842–1925), who was treating a woman named Anna O. This young woman suffered from what was then called hysteria. She experienced bouts of temporary paralysis, inability to drink water even when she was thirsty, and many other unexplainable physical conditions. Breuer found that, when hypnotized, she described situations of which she was unaware when conscious. After such sessions, her symptoms went into remission. This process became known as *the talking cure.*

In 1886, following his studies in Paris under the famous neurologist Jean-Martin Charcot (1825–1893), who also used hypnosis in studying hysteria, Freud returned to Vienna and opened his practice. Although he was still interested in the field of neurology, the nervous complaints seen in many of his wealthy female patients changed his focus. He observed that many of these complaints had no physical cause, and he concluded that they were due to what he termed *neuroses.*

Because there was no obvious cause for these neuroses, no obvious treatment was available. Freud attempted several approaches with what he called hysteric and neurotic patients, including hypnosis, which he ultimately abandoned after his discovery that patients would talk freely once they were placed in a state of relaxation. To achieve this, he had them lie on a couch and encouraged them to talk about whatever came to mind and to randomly relate early life experiences. He could then analyze the information in an effort to decipher what past traumas had induced their current mental problems. He called the process *free association*, which eventually became known as *psychoanalysis.*

Freud developed innovative and complex theories, including the concept that the psyche consists of three major divisions: the *id* (unconscious desire; instinct; repository for unfulfilled wishes and repressed thoughts unacceptable to the conscious mind), the *superego* (only partly conscious, where societal and parental rules are internalized; rewards and punishes the self through guilt, moral beliefs, and conscience), and the *ego* (the conscious mind; the mediator between the individual and his or her environment). Although these divisions of psyche are useful theoretically, there is no scientific basis for their existence. However, Freud believed that by releasing repressed, unconscious desires into the conscious through talk therapy and free association, a cure might occur.

Freud published prolifically throughout his long career, and many of his theories—especially his early ones that heavily emphasized sex—created serious controversies in the specialty. Perhaps his most controversial theories, published in 1905, were that the sex drive is stronger than any other influence in shaping an individual's psychology and that sexuality is present as early as infancy. From this base, he developed his theory of the Oedipus complex, in which young children become sexually attracted to the parent of the opposite gender and immensely jealous to the point of hating the parent of the same gender.

Another controversial theory was that of penis envy, in which, at about age 4, a girl discovers that she has no penis and suffers hurt and loss of self-esteem. Freud's work focused on the conflict between sex and moral instincts, progressed to the concept of conflict between *libido* (instinctive sex drive) and *ego*, and then to the conflict between *eros* (life instinct) and *thanatos* (death instinct). Although considered lunatic by many of his peers, Freud persisted, and in so doing he developed fascinating models of human thought and, subsequently, of human behavior: that meanings are hidden in the unconscious state of dreams, that unfulfilled wishes manifest as fantasies, that early traumatic life events, even those consciously forgotten or repressed, adversely affect the adult, along with many other models.

After being appointed professor at the University of Vienna in 1902, Freud's popularity grew, and he became surrounded by devoted followers. He and seventeen of these followers, including Alfred Adler (1870–1937) and Carl Jung (1875–1961), formed the Psychoanalytic Society, a group emulated in many other cities.

Eventually, however, political infighting caused serious disagreements among members of the group, and several once-faithful Freud followers left, some developing divergent and ultimately highly popular and influential theories in the field—Adler and Jung being two of the more famous. In Vienna and in most of Europe, Freud's theories were met with such skepticism that he was often mocked and even hated. In the less conservative West, his first international lecture series on psychoanalysis, presented at Clark University, Worcester, Massachusetts, in 1910, was a huge success. His ideas were widely espoused, his fame spread quickly across the United States, and his name became a household word. By the 1940s, psychoanalytic psychotherapy dominated the American field of psychiatry. In fact, it became virtually synonymous with the treatment of mental and emotional disturbances.

Carl Jung was a Swiss psychologist who was heavily influenced by Sigmund Freud. He split with Freud because of his disagreement with Freud's assertion that unconscious sexual repression caused all neuroses. He developed his own analytic school of psychology, and he believed in psychic phenomena, such as spiritualism, telepathy, and ESP. He also developed the metaphysical concepts of synchronicity, the collective unconscious, and archetypes.

Alfred Adler, a Viennese psychologist, was also initially heavily influenced by Freud, and he also came to disagree strongly with him. Adler moved to New York City in 1934 after developing the concept of individual psychology. He believed in a single motivating force that drives all human experience and behavior: the struggle for perfection. He is particularly well known for the theories of inferiority complex, striving for superiority, and compensation (striving to overcome). He also believed that motivation comes from being drawn toward the future through goals and ideals, whereas Freud believed that people are driven mechanically by their past.

Freud's theories were—and still are—cause for serious rifts among different psychoanalytic theorists, and many of his concepts are widely criticized for not being testable by scientific research. Regardless, Freud was undoubtedly one of the most influential scientists of the twentieth century. His theories, insights, and treatment techniques not only completely changed the professions of psychiatry, psychology, and psychotherapy, but also changed the way in which individuals—

particularly those in Western society—perceive themselves and their lives.

Description

The psychoanalytic, or psychodynamic, approach comprises two branches: psychiatry and psychology. During the early twentieth century, particularly in the United States, it became the predominant treatment modality for mental illness. This form of therapy examines the *psyche* (mind) through introspection and subjective experiences. It tends to be used primarily with people who are suffering from milder forms of mental illnesses, such as neuroses and personality disorders, and essentially healthy individuals seeking to enhance adaptive functioning. However, it is also used, often in combination with psychotropic medications, in more severe disorders, such as mood and anxiety disorders and even schizophrenia. As a treatment modality, this approach applies two basic techniques, psychoanalysis and psychotherapy, the aim of both being to help individuals understand the nature and root of their problems and to provide insight and techniques to help them cope with or overcome those problems.

Psychiatry

Psychiatry is the medical specialty that studies and treats a variety of disorders that affect the mind—mental illnesses. Because our minds create our humanity and our sense of self, our specialty cares for illnesses that affect the core of our existence.

Nancy C. Andreasen, *American Journal of Psychiatry*

The field of psychiatry is extensive and diverse, but it can be defined succinctly as the branch of medicine that researches, diagnoses, and treats mental illnesses. It is a medical specialty divided into many different subspecialties: geriatric, child, or adolescent psychiatry; mood disorders; substance and alcohol abuse; crisis intervention; psychoses; and dementias, to name just a few. Many psychiatrists practice in one subspecialty only. Once surrounded by stigma, psychiatry has grown into a legitimate discipline.

Just as cardiologists specialize in heart disease, psychiatrists specialize in disorders of the mind and brain—*mind* being mental functions, the expression of brain activity, and *brain* being the physical cells and molecules, the neurotransmitters and receptors (brain chemistry) by which mental functions are created. From its beginnings, psychiatry was divided between these two visions of mental illness. Some modern psychiatrists still focus primarily on the mind, attributing patients' problems to personal and social conditions. Others focus primarily on the brain, studying and manipulating brain anatomy and chemistry. Each, however, is studying the same thing from one of two different perspectives.

In the United States psychiatrists are specialists who, after completing 4 years of regular medical school, train as residents in the field of psychiatry for a further 4 years. They must then take written and oral examinations in order to become board certified. These examinations are so stringent that each has a failure rate of almost 50 percent. Similar requirements apply in most other countries.

Psychiatrists generally examine their patients from a biopsychosocial perspective, which may include a thorough medical examination, and they are permitted to prescribe medication. They help bring about adjustments in people's psyches through talk therapy that focuses, for example, on memories, awareness, feelings, and understanding.

Psychiatrists may also use behavioral therapy, an active, structured therapy that focuses on modifying inappropriate thoughts and, subsequently, on modifying behavior. Over time these therapies produce changes in the brain on the neuronal (cellular) level; these changes in turn affect the mind and thus thinking and behavior. Psychiatrists may treat the brain directly at the neuronal level with medications and other somatic (bodily) methods, such as electroconvulsive therapy (ECT) and psychosurgery, which in turn affect the mind and thus thoughts and behavior. In many cases, psychiatrists practice a combination of methods. With appropriate therapy, a significant number of patients find depression or anxiety lifting, hallucinations brought under control, and life regaining normalcy.

Psychiatrists treat patients either as inpatients (usually in psychiatric hospitals or in psychiatric wards in regular hospitals, where the patients may reside on a voluntary or involuntary basis), or as outpatients (people living in the normal community, who visit the psychiatrist's office periodically for anywhere from 30 to 60 minutes per visit). They treat patients with brain diseases of known causes, such as central nervous system effects of human immunodeficiency virus (HIV) infection, and with diseases of unknown causes, such as depression, anxiety, schizophrenia, and dementia.

Many psychiatrists are researchers in the neurosciences and genetics, working diligently to discover the biological causes of mental illnesses and how best to treat them and possibly to prevent them. They investigate mental deterioration in dementias as well as in normal aging, the role traumatic grief plays in triggering certain mental illnesses, and the mechanisms by which any one of the host of mental activities—imagination, introspection, memory, mood, fear, pleasure—may become disrupted, thus leading to mental illness.

Psychology

The science that deals with mental processes and behavior.
American Heritage Dictionary of the English Language

Psychology is the science of behavior, particularly of humans, but also of other animals. Like the field of psychiatry, the field of psychology is huge and diverse and divided into many subspecialties, which include health, human developmental, applied, pediatric, child, adolescent, geriatric, clinical, educational, religious, forensic, media, social, cognitive, behavioral, trauma, industrial, organizational, sports, and evolutionary psychology, as well as neuropsychology. Unlike psychiatry, which is a medical specialty, psychology is a humanistic specialty in which psychologists, therapists, and other professionals study the processes of cognition, emotion, personality, motivation, behavior, interaction between individuals, relationships, and many other aspects of an individual's existence in relation to social and environmental circumstances. The goal of psychology is to understand, predict, and modify the behavior of an individual or group.

Psychologists work in a wide variety of settings, including private practice, hospitals, schools, universities, corporations, government agencies, prisons, and legal systems. Because psychologists are not medical doctors, in the United States they are generally not permitted to prescribe medication (there are some exceptions) even though they must successfully complete and pass a licensing examination in clinical pharmacology in order to practice psychology. Many psychologists argue, therefore, that they are highly qualified to prescribe medication and should be permitted to do so.

Psychoanalysis versus Psychotherapy

Psychoanalysis: "The method of psychological therapy originated by Sigmund Freud in which free association, dream interpretation, and analysis of resistance and transference are used to explore repressed or unconscious impulses, anxieties, and internal conflicts, in order to free psychic energy for mature love and work."
American Heritage Dictionary of the English Language

Psychotherapy: "The treatment of mental and emotional disorders through the use of psychological techniques designed to encourage communication of conflicts and insight into problems, with the goal being relief of symptoms, changes in behavior leading to improved social and vocational functioning, and personality growth."
American Heritage Dictionary of the English Language

Modern psychiatry and psychology have produced a bewildering array of therapeutic modalities, each focusing on different models of mental processes (psyche) and behavior. The first model was Freudian psychoanalysis, from which psychotherapy developed. The plethora of subsequent models includes existential analysis, transactional analysis, Jungian psychotherapy, Gestalt therapy, Rogerian psychotherapy, cognitive analytic psychotherapy, neurolinguistic programming, person-centered psychotherapy, behavior therapy, cognitive behavioral therapy, encounter groups, family therapy—the list goes on. The common denominator among all these psychotherapeutic approaches is direct personal interaction between therapist and client, primarily through speech but sometimes through acting out of roles, with the ultimate goal of helping individuals deal with or solve psychosocial and behavioral problems.

BEHAVIORAL APPROACH

Brief History

Shortly after Freud introduced his psychoanalytic theories in the United States, a quite different approach to mental illness began to emerge: that of behaviorism. This approach was perhaps influenced by two earlier concepts. One was British empiricism, a school of medical practice that looked to observation, experience, and experiment for answers, while largely ignoring theory. The second was the Russian Pavlovian school, which based its psychological research on reflexes and on stimulus-response behavior. Behaviorists firmly opposed Freudian theories regarding introspection and the unconscious. They also disagreed with theories that behavior was in any way hereditary.

Perhaps most influential in the rise of behaviorism in the United States was the philosopher and psychologist John B. Watson (1878–1958), whose 1913 publication of his ideas gave birth to the behaviorist schools. Watson was born in Greenville, South Carolina. Inspired by the Russian Ivan Pavlov's (1849–1936) laboratory research using dogs as subjects, Watson studied animal behavior, biology, and physiology. He taught at the

University of Chicago, and he became professor and director of the psychological laboratory at Johns Hopkins University.

Watson also studied the behavior of children, ultimately declaring that humans and animals operated by the same basic principles. They were conditioned by experience, and they responded to situations in accordance with their *nerve pathways*. Often considered radical and extreme because of its rejection of mentalism (introspection and subjective data) and for its reduction of thought processes to conditioning and response, Watson's concept of psychology was to observe, predict, and control people's actions. One of his most influential followers was Burrhus Frederic (B. F.) Skinner (1904–1990), born in Pennsylvania, who in the 1940s began conducting research on operant learning at Harvard University using rats and pigeons as subjects. The principle behind operant learning is that there is some behavior that operates on the environment to produce a positive, reinforcing reward: for example, a rat presses a bar and is rewarded with food. Skinner was highly influential in making the behavioral model popular in the United States.

In 1920, based on his theory that children have three basic emotional reactions—fear, rage, and love—Watson and one of his graduate students, Rosalie Rayner, conducted the famous, and by modern standards highly unethical, laboratory study on an 11-month-old boy they named Little Albert to prove that children could be artificially conditioned. They determined that Little Albert responded in severe fright to a sudden loud noise. The baby also displayed amusement and interest when confronted with a white rat. Over the course of a month, Little Albert was repeatedly exposed to the loud noise just as he reached to touch the rat. Ultimately, the child was taught to be terrified of the rat. He even became afraid of other white animals, Watson's white hair, and a white Santa Claus beard. According to Watson and Rayner, all phobias develop in this way and therefore could only be treated by deconditioning, not by recovery of unconscious memories.

> Give me a dozen healthy infants, well-formed, and my own specified world to bring them up and I'll guarantee to take any one at random and train him to become any type of specialist I might select—doctor, lawyer, merchant-chief, and yes, even beggarman and thief, regardless of his talents, penchants, tendencies, abilities, vocations, and race of his ancestors.
>
> John B. Watson

Opponents rejected behaviorism as being oversimplistic and inhumane, and they claimed that the experiments were not applicable to the highly complex conditions influencing human interactions. Nevertheless, behaviorists continued to develop experiments for animals and humans to prove that behaviorism could explain all aspects of human behavior. Precise, objective, scientifically designed, carefully controlled, and based on a huge variety of behaviors, these experiments cumulatively created a convincing scientific basis for the theory of behaviorism that would, along with the psychoanalytic approach, dominate Western psychiatry until well into the second half of the twentieth century.

Description

The behavioral model is founded on the belief that the only things worth studying, or that can be scientifically studied, are things that can be seen and observed. Behaviorists therefore hold that the best way to study humans is to study what they do. Treatment primarily consists of teaching individuals how to modify their behavior, a process often referred to as conditioning. Ultimately, many schools of behaviorism developed, the basic principle espoused by each being that psychology is the natural science concerned with the objective study of behavior, with individual patterns of adjustment that are determined by responses to specific stimuli in the environment. Although this approach has been largely criticized for its lack of consideration of the motivational and cognitive factors involved in learning, the behavioral model has contributed to the pool of knowledge about how people think and why they act in certain ways, and its treatment methods can be helpful in certain mental illnesses. One highly successful and well-accepted therapeutic behavioral model is cognitive behavioral therapy (CBT).

Cognitive Behavioral Therapy
    A highly structured psychotherapeutic method used to alter distorted attitudes and problem behavior by identifying and replacing negative inaccurate thoughts and changing the rewards for behaviors.
                    American Heritage Dictionary of the English Language

CBT is a process of restructuring the mind, during which therapists, psychologists, psychiatrists, or social workers help patients to recognize automatic, irrational thought patterns and move the patient toward discovering, accepting, and employing more rational ways of thinking. This cognitive restructuring in turn creates positive behavioral changes. The ultimate goal is that rational thinking will become automatic, thus permanently encouraging positive behavior. This is a slow process, in which various methods can be employed. However, studies reveal that CBT can help people deal with many different types of problems, including substance abuse and eating disorders, mood and anxiety disorders, and, in some cases, even psychoses and schizophrenia.

THE BIOLOGICAL APPROACH

Brief History

Often referred to as the medical model, the biological approach to mental illnesses can be traced to the theories of the ancient Greeks, who asserted that mental illnesses were diseases of the mind caused by biological factors. Modern technological advances are helping neuroscientists and research psychiatrists determine with certainty that at least some mental illnesses are biologically based, arising primarily from within the brain.

While Freud was attempting to map the functions of the mind, and Watson and his followers were trying to understand the general laws governing human behavior, neuroscientists, neurologists, and some psychiatrists continued to study and map abnormalities of the brain. Perhaps the most influential of these scientists—virtually unknown in America even at the dawn of the twenty-first century but hailed throughout the rest of the world as the founding father of modern psychiatry—is the German psychiatrist Emil Kraepelin (1856–1926). During his career, Kraepelin was professor at several German medical schools and ultimately became head of the psychiatry department in Munich. There he gathered around him some of the most renowned researchers in neuroscience: Alois Alzheimer (1864–1915), for whom Alzheimer's disease was named, who microscopically identified the changes in certain brain cells that cause the disease; Franz Nissl (1860–1919), who developed a staining technique that allowed clearer observation of brain cells under the microscope; and Korbinian Brodmann (1868–1918), who used Nissl's technique to show for the first time that different sections of the brain have highly specialized functions and are composed of different types of nerve cells and thus laid the foundation for more recent and important discoveries.

As seen in the previous chapters, Kraepelin's contribution to psychiatry was to identify and describe certain types of mental illnesses. Identification and description permits diagnosis, which allows a physician to determine whether patients will improve or deteriorate, respond to a particular type of treatment, or infect others around them, or whether their children may be genetically predisposed to that illness. Kraepelin made the astounding discovery that among patients with similar symptoms, some recovered spontaneously with little treatment whereas others continued to deteriorate. Patients who experienced either euphoria accompanied by heightened energy levels or depression accompanied by greatly decreased energy levels were among the first group. Among the second group were patients whose illness manifested at a relatively young age; who suffered a wide range of symptoms, including euphoria, depression, confusion, excitement, delusions, and hallucinations; and whose slow deterioration eventually led to complete incapacitation and permanent institutionalization. The first group of symptoms he named manic-depressive insanity; the second, dementia praecox (*dementia* meaning deterioration; *praecox* meaning early age of onset). The first group is now known as *bipolar disorder*; the second, *schizophrenia*.

Kraepelin defined several other mental illnesses, and, in a series of textbooks published between 1883 and 1926, he presented careful symptom descriptions, precise case histories, and insightful hypotheses on possible causes. He hypothesized that mental illnesses were the result of some as yet unidentified physical influence—an infection or degenerative brain disease, or biological or genetic disorders—and his work became the foundation upon which modern, biologically based psychiatry is founded.

Description

The biological model emphasizes correct diagnosis through patient history, physical examination, observation of symptoms over time, and sometimes laboratory tests (primarily to identify physical illnesses that may contribute to the mental illness). Treatment emphasizes somatic therapies, primarily pharmaceutical, electroconvulsive, and, in particularly resistant cases, psychosurgical techniques. Somatic therapy—particularly medication—can affect almost miraculous alleviation of symptoms in many mental illnesses, even in more severe cases. However, no treatment is effective in all cases, and even when highly effective in controlling symptoms, treatment seldom effects a complete cure.

PSYCHOPHARMACOLOGY

Psychopharmacology is hailed by many as one of the greatest success stories in the treatment of mental illnesses and has positively affected tens of millions of individuals. It does, however, require a dedicated effort on the part of both doctor and patient: close monitoring by the doctor, and strict compliance to the recommended regimen by the patient. An overview of the major categories of psychiatric medications, including their general purpose and treatment regimen, follows. Development, mechanisms of action, and side effects are approached in the next chapter.

Antipsychotic Medications
Primary Purpose Antipsychotics, or neuroleptics, are used to treat severe emotional disorders in people who are virtually out of touch with reality: for example, those who suffer from psychotic episodes of hallucinations and delusions. These drugs revolutionized the treatment of schizophrenia and severe bipolar disorder. Antipsychotics are divided into two classes: conventional (older) and atypical (newer). They can be highly effective in lessening or eliminating many symptoms and, in some cases, shorten the course of a psychotic episode. There are dozens of brands on the market, and when one particular brand may not work for one particular patient, another may. Many antipsychotics can be taken (orally) just once a day, and some are available in "depot" forms, which are injected just once or twice a month.

Effectiveness People vary in their responses and the time it takes them to improve. Some symptoms may respond within days, some in weeks, and some in months. If little improvement occurs, a different medication may be prescribed. Some people may need to be prescribed several different medications before an effective one is found. People who have experienced one or two severe psychotic episodes will most likely need medication indefinitely, usually at a maintenance dose that is as low as possible to control symptoms, prevent relapse, and minimize side effects. In such cases, patients may decide they want to stop taking their medication, either because of unwanted side effects or because they feel they no longer need it. This will result in a disastrous return of symptoms. A partial list of antipsychotic medications appears in Table 3.1.

Antimanic Medications (Mood Stabilizers)
Primary Purpose By 2000, almost 50 percent of all people seen by psychiatrists in the United States suffered from mood disorders—among them bipolar disorder. People with bipolar disorder experience the highs of the manic cycle and the lows of the depressive cycle. Two types of drugs are used to treat this disorder: lithium, a naturally occurring salt, and anticonvulsants, commonly used to control seizures. Lithium is used most frequently, and controls or lessens the severity of the manic cycle. It

Table 3.1   Some Types of Antipsychotic Medications

Generic Name	Trade Name
Conventional	
Chlorpromazine	Thorazine
Haloperidol	Haldol
Thioridazine	Mellaril
Trifluoperazine	Stelazine
Atypical	
Clozapine	Clozaril
Quetiapine	Seroquel
Olanzapine	Zyprexa
Risperidone	Risperdal
Loxapine	Loxitane

also reduces or controls swings between cycles and is therefore used as maintenance treatment, enabling many people who would otherwise suffer from seriously incapacitating mood swings to lead normal lives. Antipsychotics are sometimes used in combination until the lithium begins to control the manic symptoms. Antidepressants are often used in combination during the depressive phase. People who experience more than one manic episode are often put on long-term maintenance treatment with lithium. For some patients, however, lithium may not help the manic phase, and others simply prefer not to take it. In such cases, anticonvulsants can be an effective alternative. Valproic acid is the anticonvulsant most often prescribed.

Effectiveness   Lithium reduces severe manic symptoms in about 5–14 days, but full control may take several weeks or months, and lithium must usually be taken for 1–2 years to achieve full benefits. Again, individual responses to treatment vary. Some people may experience no further episodes, others may experience moderate mood swings that decrease over time, and others may experience no benefit at all. However, it remains the most effective mood stabilizer for most patients who suffer from mania.

Anticonvulsants appear to be more effective in acute mania than in long-term maintenance. Some studies suggest lamotrigine is particularly effective for mania, and some suggest it is particularly effective in bipolar disorder. Valproic acid seems as effective as lithium in non–rapid-cycling bipolar disorder and more effective in rapid-cycling bipolar disorder (rapid-cycling bipolar disorder is generally defined as four or more

Table 3.2   Medications Used to Treat Mania

Generic Name	Trade Name
Lithium	
Lithium carbonate	Eskalith, Lithane, Lithobid
Lithium citrate	Cibalith-S
Anticonvulsives	
Valproic acid	Depakene, Valproate, Valrelease
Carbamazepine	Tegretol
Divalproex sodium (valproic acid)	Depakote
Gabapentin	Neurontin
Lamotrigine	Lamictal

distinct episodes of mania/hypomania and depression or mixed episodes in 1 year, with periods of normal mood between episodes).

Other types of medication are often prescribed in combination to treat accompanying symptoms of agitation, anxiety, insomnia, or depression, and finding the most effective medication or combination of medications proves to be worthwhile. Antimanic medications are listed in Table 3.2.

Antidepressant Medications

Primary Purpose   Antidepressants are most frequently used to treat major depressive illnesses and bipolar disorder, are sometimes prescribed for milder forms of depression, and are often used in combination with antianxiety medication to treat extreme anxiety. For people who have experienced one or two depressive episodes, medication may be necessary for a relatively short period only—perhaps 6–12 months. For those severely or continually depressed or who experience frequent recurring bouts, antidepressants may be required over the long term or even for life. Antidepressants fall into three major categories: tricyclics, monoamine oxidase inhibitors (MAOIs), and the more modern selective serotonin reuptake inhibitors (SSRIs). Mirtazapine, venlafaxine, trazodone, and bupropion are independent of the three classes. Tricyclics are sometimes used for several other mental illnesses and conditions, such as the following:

- Bulimia (eating disorder)
- Attention deficit hyperactivity disorder (ADHD)
- Narcolepsy (extreme tendency to fall asleep suddenly)
- Smoking cessation
- Panic disorder
- Urinary incontinence

Table 3.3   A Partial List of Medications Used to Treat Depression

Generic Name	Brand Name
Tricyclics	
Amitriptyline	Elavil
Imipramine	Tofranil
Doxepin	Adapin, Sinequan
SSRIs	
Citalopram	Celexa
Fluoxetine	Prozac
Paroxetine	Paxil
Sertraline	Zoloft
MAOIs	
Isocarboxazid	Marplan
Phenelzine	Nardil
Tranylcypromine	Parnate
Others	
Bupropion	Wellbutrin
Venlafaxine	Effexor
Mirtazapine	Remeron
Trazodone	Desyrel

Effectiveness   Depression can be severely debilitating and is a major cause of suicide, and antidepressants can be a highly effective form of treatment. It may be 1 or 2 weeks after initiation of treatment before patients begin to feel the benefit of antidepressants, but it will most likely be 6–8 weeks before full benefits are felt. Several different brands may have to be prescribed before one is found for which a benefit is felt, but most patients will respond to one of these medications. Dosage varies with type of drug and an individual's characteristics. In resistant cases, an additional medication, such as lithium, may be necessary. MAOIs can also be effective in resistant cases. There are more than two dozen different types of antidepressants available. A partial list is found in Table 3.3.

Antianxiety Medications

Primary Purpose   Extreme and prolonged anxiety is serious and can make activities of daily living virtually impossible. Antianxiety medications can be extremely effective. Some antidepressants, including MAOIs, may also be helpful. Only two classes of antianxiety medications have to

Table 3.4   Antianxiety Medications. All Except Buspirone
            (BuSpar) are Benzodiazepines

Generic Name	Brand Name
Alprazolam	Xanax
Buspirone	BuSpar
Chlordiazepoxide	Librax, Libritabs, Librium
Clonazepam	Klonopin
Clorazepate	Azene, Tranxene
Diazepam	Valium
Halazepam	Paxipam
Lorazepam	Ativan
Oxazepam	Serax
Prazepam	Centrax

date been developed specifically to treat anxiety: benzodiazepines and a member of the azaperone class called buspirone, which is usually prescribed for generalized anxiety disorders (GAD). Depending on the patient's condition, antianxiety drugs may be taken two or three times a day, once a day, or even on an "as-needed" basis. Beta blockers, usually prescribed for high blood pressure and heart conditions, may be prescribed to alleviate "performance anxiety" when an individual must face a particularly stressful situation.

Effectiveness   Benzodiazepines usually work quickly, whereas buspirone must be taken as prescribed for a minimum of 2 weeks before positive effects are obvious and is thus not used on an as-needed basis. A list of antianxiety medications is shown in Table 3.4.

Because many mental illnesses are believed to be caused by a combination of biological, psychological, and sociological factors and because they affect virtually every aspect of an individual's life, patients who are treated primarily with medication often benefit greatly from combining it with psychotherapy.

ELECTROCONVULSIVE THERAPY

Primary Purpose

ECT, often known as electric shock therapy, is used to treat people with severe depression that is nonresponsive to medication and/or psychotherapy, particularly when accompanied by suicidal tendencies. It is also sometimes used to treat mania. ECT involves applying a small electric current to the brain to produce seizure-like activity. The patient is first sedated and given muscle relaxants, which prevent the violent muscle contractions that can occur during the induced seizures. Treatments are individualized, but generally are given three times a week for a total of four to eight treatments.

Effectiveness
Alleviation of depressive symptoms occurs quickly, and this treatment is reported to be effective in approximately 80 percent of cases. However, controversy remains as to how long the treatment remains effective and the rates of relapse.

PSYCHOSURGERY

Primary Purpose
Psychosurgery is used as a last resort to treat behavior, personality, obsessive-compulsive (OCD), and bipolar disorders, and severe depression nonresponsive to all other forms of treatment. During psychosurgery, certain areas of the brain are disabled by severing or otherwise destroying connective nerve fibers or tissue in certain pathways that connect the frontal cortex (where thought processes originate) and the limbic system (where it is believed emotions are seated). One such procedure was the lobotomy, which has since been replaced by other major procedures, four of which are anterior cingulotomy, subcaudate tractotomy, limbic leukotomy, and capsulotomy.

Effectiveness
Historically, determining the effectiveness of psychosurgery has been extremely difficult. However, several studies over the last three decades of the twentieth century have reported on several different psychosurgical methods:

> *Anterior cingulotomy*: Studies show that approximately 25–30 percent of patients achieved at least a 35 percent improvement in symptoms.
> *Anterior capsulotomy*: Improvement in OCD is reported in 70 percent of patients; comparisons indicate a higher efficacy rate than with anterior cingulotomy.
> *Subacute tractotomy*: In a 1970 study, depression or anxiety was reported to improve in two out of three patients and OCD in approximately 50 percent of patients. A study conducted between 1979 and 1991 of 249 patients indicated an approximately 34 percent positive treatment response.

Limbic leukotomy: A 2002 Massachusetts General Hospital study indicated a 36–50 percent positive response rate in patients with OCD or major depressive disorder. Four of five patients suffering OCD or schizoaffective disorder accompanied by self-mutilation showed reduction in destructive behavior, and two out of three showed reduced assaultive tendencies.

BARRIERS TO TREATMENT OF MENTAL ILLNESSES

As already noted, one in five Americans (approximately 20 percent) suffer from a mental illness, yet the majority of those who need it do not seek treatment, even though in many instances mental illnesses are highly treatable. Reasons for not seeking treatment include the following:

- Stigma
- High cost of treatment
- Fear of disclosure by physicians or insurance companies to family or employer
- Fear of being hospitalized
- Belief by the individual that the illness can be handled without treatment
- Belief by the individual that no one can help
- Lack of personal awareness of having a mental illness, especially in those with a severe illness such as schizophrenia
- Demographic factors: African Americans, Hispanics, and poor white women are less likely than non-Hispanic whites to seek treatment
- Significantly underestimated prevalence of mental health problems among children

Two of the greatest barriers to treatment are stigma and the high cost of treatment.

Stigma

Stigma is the primary barrier to treatment. Many people with mental disorders feel too ashamed or embarrassed to seek treatment because public perception has long been distorted by untruths and ignorance. Mental illness was at one time (and by the uninformed is still) blamed on the individual, who was accused of being either personally or spiritually flawed. In mainstream media and the modern entertainment industry, violence, aggression, and unpredictable behavior is often attributed to mental illness. Jokes; degrading terminology, such as "lunatic," "psycho," and "retarded";

and distorted, negative images still abound. The media generally covers mental illness in relation to violent crimes and excludes it from the type of sensitive coverage given to other illnesses, such as cancer, diabetes, and cardiac disease. This negative attention continues and reinforces old stereotypes, misunderstandings, and inaccuracies. The following are just some of the negative effects of stigmatization:

- Discrimination by insurance agencies, which severely limit and even deny coverage for any form of mental illness
- Violence, mistrust, and fear toward the mentally ill and their families
- Prejudice and discrimination in many forms, including employment, education, and housing
- Rejection by friends and family

When someone appears to be different than us, we may view him or her in a negative stereotyped manner. People who have identities that society values negatively are said to be stigmatized. Stigma is a reality for people with a mental illness, and they report that how others judge them is one of their greatest barriers to a complete and satisfying life.

Canadian Mental Health Association

The media has come a long way in showing minorities, women, mentally retarded individuals, and gay persons in a much more honest and truthful light. It's about time they did the same for people with mental illness.

Kurt Douglass Sass, *New York City Voices*, April/May 2002

Cost of Treatment

Another negative effect of stigma and a huge barrier to treatment is the cost of treatment, whether by psychoactive medication or psychotherapy. Either way, treatment is expensive, and in 2004, 37 million people in the United States lived in poverty, and 45.8 million—and increase of 800,000 from 2003—had no medical insurance. Even people with insurance most likely have less comprehensive coverage for mental illnesses than for physical illnesses, because most policies discriminate between the two. Insurance policies exclude or severely limit support for psychiatric treatment by imposing higher deductibles and copayments, lower annual and lifetime limits, and fewer days of hospitalization or outpatient visitations. Prescription coverage for psychiatric medications is also usually severely reduced, restricted, or even denied entirely.

CHAPTER 4

Scientific Discoveries and Advances: Twentieth-Century Developments

The 1930s saw the dawn of modern scientific methods to treat mental illness: insulin shock therapy that induced temporary coma to treat schizophrenia, electroconvulsive therapy (ECT), and psychosurgery. Of these original techniques, the first is no longer practiced. Especially important for the treatment of mental illness was the development of psychopharmacology. Finally, two other developments, brain imaging and the mapping of the human genome, brought about exciting possibilities for understanding, treating, and hopefully preventing mental illness.

ELECTROCONVULSIVE THERAPY

ECT, which involves delivering electrical currents to the head to activate the brain and induce mild seizures, is believed by many psychiatrists to be an effective therapy for severely and suicidally depressed patients who are otherwise unresponsive to treatment. Its crude beginnings and its introduction into American hospitals date to the 1940s, but its severe effects, which were often physically and mentally damaging, its overuse, and its abuse eventually brought it into serious disrepute. ECT is now done under anesthesia with the use of muscle relaxants to prevent the bone breaks and fractures once caused by the induced seizures. Proponents claim it has developed into a highly sophisticated and safe treatment modality, and approximately 100,000 people in the United States are treated with it annually.

Side Effects

The most significant side effect of modern ECT is short-term memory loss, which may worsen as the number of treatments increases. This problem usually resolves over the several weeks after treatment ends, and although hotly disputed by some, others believe there is no significant evidence of long-term memory loss in patients treated with ECT.

PSYCHOSURGERY

Psychosurgery was initially commonly called *lobotomy*. In the United States alone, an estimated 20,000–50,000 people were operated on between 1936 and the mid-1950s. Due to indiscriminate use, the danger involved, and the often irreversible, debilitating results, it eventually fell from favor. By the dawn of the twenty-first century, however, a refined set of psychosurgical techniques, consisting of four different procedures, was being used in especially difficult cases: anterior cingulotomy, anterior capsulotomy, subacute tractotomy, and limbic leukotomy.

Side Effects

Permanent brain damage is the most serious risk factor associated with psychosurgery. Noninvasive techniques using stereotactic radiosurgery, including the gamma knife (a noninvasive surgical tool that focuses radiation beams at the head, which converge at the targeted site in the brain to create a lesion there) have significantly reduced that risk. Although disputed by some, others believe that there appears to be little postsurgical memory loss or loss of other high-level cognitive processes. Risk factors for the four procedures include the following:

Anterior cingulotomy: exacerbated urinary incontinence, medically responsive seizures, risk of postoperative epilepsy.

Anterior capsulotomy: confusion, weight gain, depression, nocturnal incontinence, cognitive and affective dysfunction, decreased initiative and drive. In 1999, a group of psychiatrists from the Karolinska Institute in Sweden indicated that these adverse effects appear to normalize in the long term.

Subacute tractotomy: immediate and longer-term side effects seem to occur more frequently than with cingulotomy, and include seizures and negative personality traits.

Limbic leukotomy: transient adverse effects.

PSYCHOPHARMACOLOGY

Psychopharmacology, which began in earnest in the 1950s, is perhaps one of the greatest success stories and remarkable advancements in the treatment of mental illnesses. Psychotherapeutic medications have significantly improved the lives of tens of millions of people suffering from mental illnesses. Not only do such medications have a direct effect of alleviating symptoms, in so doing, they can make other forms of therapy more effective. For example, a patient in psychotherapy may be so severely depressed that communication is virtually impossible. Appropriate medication may alleviate depression enough that the individual can engage in productive talk or behavioral therapy, thus increasing chances of a permanent cure. Also, psychotherapeutic medication has helped researchers better understand how the brain works and what type of biochemical malfunctions cause some mental illnesses.

Many drugs initially used in treating mental illnesses were developed for other purposes, and their psychotherapeutic value was discovered by accident. By the close of the twentieth century, radically increased understanding of brain function and chemistry enabled a far more scientific approach to the development of new drugs. Looking forward, research psychiatrists are optimistic that identifying molecular and genetic causes of specific mental illnesses will enable the development of even more highly targeted drugs.

Mechanisms of Action: How Drugs Work

Although the mechanisms of action of psychotropic drugs are not definitively known, they are believed—and a growing body of research evidence supports the hypothesis—to interact with chemicals in the brain called *neurotransmitters*.

Brain Chemistry: Electrical Signals and Neurotransmitters   The brain functions through the action of nerve cells called *neurons*—somewhere around 100 billion of them. Neurons are highly complex communication centers that pass electrical and chemical signals between each other. Simplistically described, neurons are cell bodies from which nerve fibers extend. These fibers are called *axons* and *dendrites*. An axon is the pathway through which the cell body sends electrical signals, and dendrites help the cell receive messages from other cells. Each cell usually has only one axon, the end of which branches out into many terminals where chemicals called *neurotransmitters* are stored in tiny vesicles (sacs). The junction at which signals are transmitted from one cell to the next, via the axon of the sender to the dendrites of the receiver, is called a *synapse*. Membranes surrounding the terminals on the cell sending the signal are called *presynaptic* membranes and membranes surrounding dendrites on the cell receiving the signal are called *postsynaptic* membranes. Pre- and postsynaptic membranes are separated by a tiny space called the *synaptic gap*. Because the electrical signal emitted by the sending cell cannot jump this gap, the signal instead stimulates and releases neurotransmitters from the presynaptic vesicles. The neurotransmitters then enter the gap and are received by the postsynaptic membranes of the receiving cell, which contain *receptors*—large protein molecules that recognize specific neurotransmitters. Neurotransmitters fit into their matching receptors like pairs of matching pieces in a puzzle. However, not all the released neurotransmitter enters the receiving cell, and leftover neurotransmitters circulate freely around the cells. The receiving cell responds to the neurotransmitters by firing off an appropriate electrical current, which in turn travels along its axon and releases neurotransmitters from its presynaptic vesicles to communicate with the next cell. Diagrams of these mechanisms are shown in Figures 4.1 and 4.2.

An intricate balance of the numerous neurotransmitters is required for the brain to function properly, and an optimal balance is maintained by proteins called *enzymes*. Enzymes regulate the amount of neurotransmitters circulating in the brain by breaking down and removing about 10 percent of the excess. Other excess neurotransmitters are taken back into the cell that released it in a process called *reuptake*. Once reuptake occurs, the neurotransmitter no longer affects the brain. A disruption in

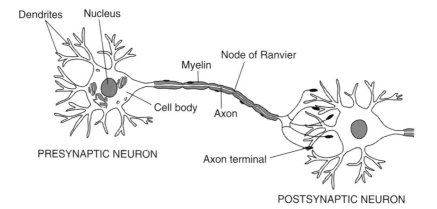

Figure 4.1
Pathways of electrochemical signaling between cells. (Ricochet Productions.)

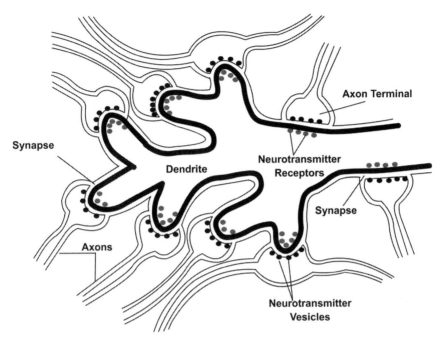

Figure 4.2
The synapse, where information is exchanged between cells. (Ricochet Productions.)

either of these processes can cause an imbalance of neurotransmitters, and this is believed to be the cause of many mental illnesses. Common neurotransmitters believed to be associated with mental illnesses are shown in Table 4.1.

Development of Psychiatric Drugs

Antimanics, or Mood Stabilizers   One of the earliest psychoactive drugs, used primarily to treat mania in bipolar disorder, is lithium. In the second century, Greek physician Soranus of Ephesus (c. 98–138) recommended that people suffering from mania be treated with the alkaline waters in his town that contained high levels of lithium salts. The rediscovery of lithium by Australian psychiatrist John Cade in the 1940s as an effective treatment for symptoms of manic depression (bipolar disorder) was an important event. Originally used as a salt substitute, lithium was found by Cade to have sedating effect on psychotic patients; however, lithium treatment was not adopted until the 1960s, when systematic studies by the Danish psychiatrist Mogens Schou found it to be effective in treating

**Table 4.1   Some Common Neurotransmitters, Their Functions, and
Their Effects**

Transmitter	What it seems to do	Problems if it gets out of balance
Serotonin or 5-HT	In the body, 5-HT is involved with blood pressure and gut control. In the brain, it controls mood, emotions, sleep/wake, feeding, temperature regulation, etc.	Too much serotonin and you feel sick, less hungry, get headaches or migraines. Too little and you feel depressed, drowsy, etc.
Dopamine —there are three main groups (or pathways) of dopamine neurones in the brain	In the brain, one group controls muscle tension and another controls, e.g., emotions, perceptions, sorting out what is real/important/imaginary, etc.	Not enough dopamine in the first group and your muscles tighten up (e.g., as in Parkinson's Disease). Too much dopamine in the second group gives you an overactive brain, i.e., too much "perception," e.g., you may see, hear, or imagine things that are not real.
Noradrenaline (NA) (sometimes called "norepinephrine" or NE)	In the body, it controls the heart and blood pressure. In the brain, it controls sleep, wakefulness, arousal, mood, emotion, and drive.	Too much noradrenaline and you may feel anxious, jittery, etc. Too little and you may feel depressed, sedated, dizzy, have low blood pressure, etc.
Acetylcholine (ACh)	In the body, acetylcholine passes the messages which make muscles contract. In the brain, it controls arousal, the ability to use memory, learning tasks, etc.	Too much in your body and your muscles tighten up. Too little can produce dry mouth, blurred vision, and constipation, as well as becoming confused, drowsy, slow at learning, etc.
Glutamate	Acts as an "accelerator" in the brain.	Too much and you become anxious, excited, and some parts of your brain may become overactive.
GABA	Acts as a "brake" in the brain.	Too little and you may become drowsy or sedated. Too little and you may become anxious and excited.

Source: Norfolk and Waveney Mental Health Partnership NHS Trust.

mania and stabilizing, over the long term, the extreme mood swings in manic depression. By 1970, lithium was being used to treat affective disorders, including bipolar disorder, for which it became—and remains— the most effective mood stabilizer available.

Mechanism of Action   Lithium's mechanism of action is complex and not well understood; however, one promising theory is that lithium suppresses inositol monophosphate signaling involved in the second-messenger system, a biochemical pathway inside the cells that contributes to cell action and is activated by first messengers, such as neurotransmitters. Another theory is that it has long-term effects on gene transcription (the process by which the DNA in a gene is read, triggering a response that creates proteins) and the regulation of G protein actions, thus altering (modulating) the behavior of certain neurotransmitter receptors.

Side Effects   At first, people may experience uncomfortable side effects, among which are the following:

- Drowsiness
- Weakness
- Nausea
- Fatigue
- Hand tremor
- Dry mouth, and increased thirst and urination
- Weight gain
- Hypothyroidism (underactive thyroid)
- Confusion

Lithium may cause birth defects, and it is present in mothers' milk. At higher levels, muscle twitches, increased drowsiness, confusion, fits, and even unconsciousness may occur. Some side effects may eventually decrease or disappear altogether, although hand tremors may continue. Lithium can interact negatively with many other medications, and its use requires regular monitoring and strict compliance.

Anticonvulsants   Certain anticonvulsant drugs used primarily to treat epilepsy, including carbamazepine (Tegretol), valproic acid (Valproate, Depakene, Valrelease), and clonazepam (Klonopin), can be effective mood-stabilizing adjuncts to lithium in treating rapid-cycling bipolar disorder, which is generally defined as four or more distinct episodes of mania/hypomania and depression or mixed episodes in 1 year, with periods of normal mood between episodes.

Mechanism of Action   Exactly how these medications work as mood stabilizers remains uncertain.

Side Effects   Valproic acid can cause gastrointestinal side effects; however, the incidence of these is low. It is known to have caused liver dysfunction, and liver function tests are recommended before and at frequent intervals during the first 6 months of therapy in particular. Other side effects of anticonvulsants include the following:

- Headache
- Double vision
- Dizziness
- Anxiety
- Confusion

Antipsychotics   Symptoms of schizophrenia can be significantly alleviated by antipsychotics, also known as *neuroleptics*. Perhaps the most significant event in the treatment of mental illness was the discovery in the mid-1950s of the antipsychotic chlorpromazine (Thorazine), the first drug used in the treatment of mental illness. Initially developed as an antihistamine and called promethazine, the antipsychotic action of chlorpromazine was discovered virtually by accident. It caused an undesirable sedating effect, and in 1952, in an effort to calm their psychiatric patients, the French psychiatrists Jean Delay and Pierre Deniker experimented with the drug on many of their patients, including those with mania, depression, and schizophrenia. They discovered that, apart from its potent calming effect, it drastically decreased hallucinations and delusional thoughts, yet allowed the patient to remain mentally alert.

For the first time in history, psychiatry had a drug that alleviated the devastating symptoms of schizophrenia, and many patients who had been hospitalized for years could function well enough to live independently and receive the necessary care in community settings. Until the early 1950s, half of all hospital beds around the world encompassing all types of physical and mental illnesses were occupied by people with schizophrenia. Between 1950 and 1970, due in part to the development of chlorpromazine, the number of patients in mental institutions alone dropped by 50 percent.

Conventional, or Typical, Antipsychotics   Lithium, the "wonder drug," can have serious and devastating adverse side effects on some patients, some of whom refused to take it, preferring, instead, to suffer with their disorder. Consequently, researchers around the world began developing a plethora of other drugs in hopes of finding other antipsychotic agents. This indeed occurred, and *conventional* or *typical* antipsychotics, such as haloperidol (Haldol), thioridazine (Mellaril), and others, became popular.

Mechanisms of Action   Conventional antipsychotics work solely by binding to and blocking dopamine D_2 receptors on cells in the brain's mesolimbic pathway (involved in the control of memory and emotion), thus preventing D_2 neurotransmitter activity.

Side Effects   Dopamine also plays an important role in controlling muscle movement, and because conventional antipsychotics bind to D_2 receptors in parts of the brain other than the mesolimbic pathway, they cause *extrapyramidal side effects* (EPS) that range from mildly unpleasant to severe and potentially debilitating, such as:

- Parkinson's-like symptoms, including muscle rigidity and tremors
- Dystonia, characterized by painful, severe, and sustained muscle contractions that in many cases are transient but are persistent in 1.5–2 percent of individuals; this is known as *tardive dystonia*
- Akathisia, which manifests in extreme restlessness and jittery movements
- Tardive dyskinesia, represented by involuntary facial movements, sucking and chewing, lip smacking, tongue twisting, and often purposeless and jerky limb movements
- Neuroleptic malignant syndrome, very rare but potentially fatal, in which movement disorders associated with EPS are accompanied by an extremely high fever

Although these medications, including chlorpromazine (Thorazine), reduce hallucinations and delusions (*positive* symptoms), they have little or no effect on lethargy, lack of emotion, lack of interest, or inability to think fluidly (*negative* symptoms). Therefore, although many patients with schizophrenia improved, they were by no means well. More would be needed.

Atypical Antipsychotics   In the 1990s, several new drugs for schizophrenia, commonly known as *next-generation* or *atypical* antipsychotics because they not only control positive symptoms but also improve negative symptoms and have significantly reduced side effects, became available. The first, clozapine, was developed and used in Europe, but was virtually abandoned because it reduces white blood cells (which fight infection) to a dangerous level, causing a serious blood disorder known as agranulocytosis. However, American psychiatrists John Kane and Herbert Meltzer tested it on patients unresponsive to other antipsychotics and closely monitored blood counts to prevent agranulocytosis. The drug proved highly effective, and many chronically ill patients improved significantly.

Paul Janssen, who developed the first-generation antipsychotic haloperidol, synthesized another new and successful drug called risperidone. This drug targeted receptors for other neurotransmitters besides dopamine and required no blood monitoring. The development of other neuroleptics soon followed—aripiprazole (Abilify), olanzapine (Zyprexa), quetiapine (Seroquel), and ziprasidone (Geodon)—which appeared to be better tolerated than the first-generation drugs, although this claim is in dispute. Clozapine, however, remains the treatment of choice for people whose symptoms are difficult to treat.

Mechanism of Action   The mechanism of action of atypical antipsychotics is more complex than that of conventional antipsychotics, as they do not exclusively affect dopamine D_2 receptors. Clozapine, for example, interacts with D_2, serotonin (5-HT), and noradrenaline (NE) receptors, and risperidone acts on D_2, serotonin type 2 (5-HT$_2$), H-1 histamine, and a1 adrenergic receptors.

Side Effects   Each atypical drug has specific side effects. They were initially thought to be far less likely to cause EPS than the first-generation drugs, but a 2003 meta-analysis of a number of studies brought that assumption into question. Common side effects for atypical antipsychotics include the following:

- Dizziness
- Drowsiness
- Headaches
- Hormonal disturbances causing sexual dysfunction
- Impaired cognitive function
- Photosensitivity
- Rapid heartbeat
- Short-term gastrointestinal symptoms and nausea
- Occasionally, feelings of unreality and depersonalization, usually short-lived

Antidepressants and Mood Stabilizers   Medications to treat mood disorders fall into one of two classes: antidepressants and mood stabilizers. Mood disorders, often called affective disorders, are characterized by either depression, mania, or a combination of both—the latter is known as bipolar disorder. Perhaps one of the greatest success stories in modern psychiatry in particular and modern medicine in general is the discovery of medication to treat mood disorders. Each antidepressant has its unique side (or adverse) effects, but most side effects are temporary and typically not serious.

Tricyclic Antidepressants   In the 1950s, hot on the heels of chlorpromazine, came another major breakthrough. By slightly changing the chemical structure of chlorpromazine in an attempt to create a better antipsychotic drug, a Swiss chemical company produced a new substance that they named imipramine and that had similar calming effects to chlorpromazine. Using it on schizophrenic patients, Swiss psychiatrist Roland Kuhn discovered that although its effect on hallucinations and delusions was slight, symptoms of depression improved. Experiments on depressed patients often brought about remarkable improvement. This subsequently became the first in a new class of drugs called *tricyclic* antidepressants—tricyclic because their chemical structure consists of three rings. By the mid-1950s, a number of different tricyclic antidepressants were available. Among the most widely used are imipramine, amitriptyline, desipramine, nortriptyline, protriptyline, doxepin, and clomipramine. Due to their high rate of success in treating depression, they became extensively used throughout the world.

Mechanisms of Action   Tricyclics increase the levels of norepinephrine, dopamine, and serotonin circulating in the brain by inhibiting their reuptake.

Side Effects   Tricyclics have a highly lethal cardiotoxic effect in overdose situations. Other common side effects include the following:

- Dry mouth
- Constipation
- Bladder problems
- Sexual dysfunction
- Blurred vision
- Dizziness upon rising or standing up
- Daytime drowsiness
- Elevated heart rate

Monoamine Oxidase Inhibitors   Also around the 1950s, a third class of drugs was developed: monoamine oxidase inhibitors, commonly known as

MAOIs. As indicated by their name, these medications work by inhibiting production of the neurotransmitter monoamine oxidase. Again, their application to mental illnesses occurred virtually by accident. The initial drug, iproniazid, was developed as an antibiotic to treat tuberculosis. However, astute and observant clinicians noticed that it had a positive effect on symptoms of mental illness. This drug, too, was tested on a wide range of psychiatric patients and was found to alleviate depression. Subsequently, more effective MAOIs were developed, particularly isocarboxazid (Marplan), phenelzine (Nardil), and tranylcypromine (Parnate). Although somewhat less effective in general than other antidepressants, MAOIs have less unpleasant side effects, but due to serious and possibly fatal interactions with certain foods, drinks, and medications, both physicians and patients are often reluctant to use them. Prescribed and taken responsibly, however, the drugs are safe, and because they are often effective where other antidepressants fail, they became the second-line treatment for depression.

Mechanism of Action   MAOIs increase levels of norepinephrine, dopamine, and serotonin by inhibiting production of monoamine oxidase, the enzyme responsible for degrading (destroying) them. They also have an effect on tyramine levels, a molecule involved in regulating blood pressure.

Side Effects   Serious and potentially fatal adverse effects can occur between MAOIs and food and beverages containing high levels of tyramine, as well as with many medications, including the following:

- Aged cheeses
- Wines, particularly red wines, and other alcoholic beverages
- Pickles
- Other antidepressants and prescription medications
- Over-the-counter drugs, including cold medicines and antihistamines
- Certain herbal supplements
- Street drugs

Selective Serotonin Reuptake Inhibitors   In the 1990s, a new class of drugs known as "new-generation" antidepressants hit the market, collectively called *selective serotonin reuptake inhibitors* (SSRIs). Developed in the early 1980s, these drugs offered new hope to people suffering from depression, panic disorder, obsessive-compulsive behavior, and similar disorders. Recognizing that some of the older antidepressants worked on the neurotransmitter serotonin, certain drug companies began developing drugs to selectively affect reuptake of serotonin, from which their name arises.

First came fluoxetine (Prozac), which immediately became popular and remains so. Others, such as paroxetine (Paxil), sertraline (Zoloft), citalopram (Celexa), and fluvoxamine (Luvox), soon followed. They are highly effective in many instances but have also been blamed for violent behavior, homicide, and suicide, particularly in children and adolescents. As of 2006, certain brands remained the subject of considerable controversy.

Mechanism of Action　　Among its many actions, the neurotransmitter serotonin has an antidepressant function. SSRIs inhibit reuptake of serotonin, allowing more of the neurotransmitter to circulate through the brain.

Side Effects　　SSRIs are potentially lethal when taken with MAOIs. They have been blamed for violent acts and suicide. Common side effects include the following:

- Sexual dysfunction
- Headache
- Nausea
- Nervousness, difficulty falling asleep, or waking frequently at night
- Agitation

Mixed-Action Antidepressants　　Mixed-action antidepressants, such as venlafaxine (Effexor), bupropion (Wellbutrin), mirtazapine (Remeron), and nefazodone (Serzone), fall into none of the previous classes and appear to cause fewer serious side effects, particularly sexual dysfunction; however, the long-term effects of these drugs remain unknown.

Mechanism of Action　　Although the mechanism of action of these medications is not well understood, they ultimately appear to act similarly to tricyclics and SSRIs, increasing the amounts of serotonin and/or norepinephrine circulating in the brain.

Side Effects　　Wellbutrin has been reported to cause seizures and sometimes death, with risks increasing with higher doses. The most common side effects of mixed-action antidepressants include the following:

- Weight loss
- Increased/decreased appetite
- Ringing in the ears
- Agitation/anxiety
- Rapid heartbeat
- Dry mouth

- Insomnia
- Headache
- Nausea and vomiting
- Constipation
- Tremors
- Drowsiness or difficulty sleeping

Antianxiety Agents   Still another class of drugs was developed in the 1950s: tranquilizers. Barbiturates such as phenobarbital were the first type of drug used to treat anxiety, but they proved to be highly sedative and addictive. In 1954, a new tranquilizing agent known as meprobamate, developed by the Czech scientist Frank Berger, was introduced and marketed as Equanil and Miltown. Although effective in treating anxiety, at first seemingly without the negative side effects of barbiturates, it, too, caused serious dependency and was highly lethal in suicide attempts. However, it set the stage for development of newer tranquilizers, which were eventually renamed *antianxiety agents*: the benzodiazepines. The large number of benzodiazepines includes chlordiazepoxide (Librium), diazepam (Valium), lorazepam (Ativan), and alprazolam (Xanax). Buspirone (BuSpar), which is not a benzodiazepine, is the only other drug specifically used to treat anxiety, although many antidepressants are also effective for anxiety disorders. The first medication specifically approved for treating obsessive-compulsive disorder (OCD)—classified as an anxiety disorder—was the tricyclic antidepressant clomipramine (Anafranil). Some new-generation antidepressants—fluoxetine, fluvoxamine, paroxetine, and sertraline—are approved for treating OCD; sertraline is also approved for post-traumatic stress disorder (PTSD) and panic disorder; paroxetine for panic disorder, generalized anxiety disorder (GAD) and social anxiety disorder; and venlafaxine (Effexor) for GAD.

Mechanism of Action   Benzodiazepines appear to be gamma-aminobutyric acid (GABA) agonists, which means they enhance the effect of that neurotransmitter. GABA is an inhibitory neurochemical, producing a quieting effect on the brain. Benzodiazepines, therefore, enhance this influence, producing muscle-relaxing and sedative effects. Buspirone, on the other hand, does not affect GABA receptors, but is thought to be a partial serotonin agonist, thus increasing the amounts of that neurochemical in the brain.

Side Effects   *Benzodiazepines*: Tolerance, dependence, and abuse can occur with long-term use of benzodiazepines, and withdrawal difficulties are possible, some of which actually mimic the anxiety state. They are therefore usually prescribed for short periods only. Interaction with alcohol and some medications can cause serious and potentially life-threatening complications. Generally, however, they have relatively few side effects, the most common being the following:

- Loss of coordination
- Drowsiness
- Fatigue
- Mental slowness
- Confusion

Buspirone: Possible side effects include dizziness, headaches, and nausea.

BRAIN IMAGING

As the twentieth century drew to a close, technological advances had opened up a bright new era of research. Scientists and psychiatrists could now observe the activity of the brain and study genes. The first important tool was the electroencephalogram (EEG), which measures electrical activity in the brain. Computed tomography (CT), which became available in the mid-1970s, later allowed researchers to noninvasively image, and therefore visualize and measure, brain function. Other imaging techniques quickly followed: magnetic resonance imaging (MRI), single photon emission CT (SPECT), and positron emission tomography (PET), which allows visualization of the brain while it is actually functioning to generate the mind.

Differences in brain function between people with and without mental illness could now be observed, and structural abnormalities were discovered in patients with certain mental illnesses, including schizophrenia (Figure 4.3), some mood disorders, alcoholism, Alzheimer's disease and other forms of dementia, and anorexia nervosa. Brain imaging provided scientific evidence that mental illnesses arise in the brain, and although as of 2006 it could not be used for diagnosis or screening, scientists could nevertheless better see how nerve cells communicate and how certain drugs block certain chemical receptors or neurotransmitters, allowing more accurate doses of medication to be determined and thus avoiding many unwanted side effects.

GENOMICS

The parallel investigations into the human genome brought another major breakthrough in the understanding of mental illnesses. In 1953, American James Watson and British Francis Crick at last uncovered the structure of deoxyribose nucleic acid (DNA), which contains all the genetic information necessary to create a new organism. The human genome is made up of approximately 20,000–25,000 genes located on the DNA molecules. DNA molecules are organized into twenty-three

SCHIZOPHRENIA IN IDENTICAL TWINS

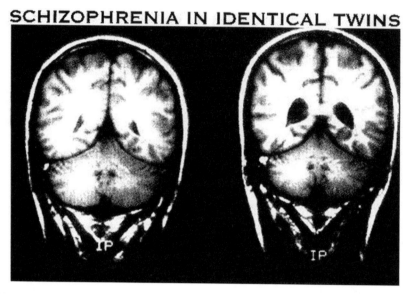

Figure 4.3
Picture of 28-year-old identical twins, one with schizophrenia and the other well. It clearly illustrates two points: (1) schizophrenia is a brain disease with measurable structural and functional abnormalities in the brain; and (2) it is not purely a genetic disease, and other factors play a role in its etiology. (Courtesy of Drs. E. Fuller Torrey and Daniel Weinberger.)

pairs of chromosomes. All twenty-three pairs of chromosomes are located in the nucleus of almost every one of the trillions of cells in the human body (see Figure 4.4). By mid-2000, a full century of scientific study and research had resulted in the mapping of 97 percent of the human genome, an undertaking that was 99 percent complete by 2003.

As early as 1996, however, scientists had found evidence that bipolar disorder may be linked to certain chromosomes. A large study completed in 1997 determined that it was linked to at least six and possibly more chromosomes, and a 2001 study indicated chromosome 22 may be specifically involved. Research thus indicates a hereditary, or genetic, predisposition (likelihood) to the disorder. Similar studies indicate a genetic predisposition to schizophrenia and to severe depression. Although by 2006 no genetic test was as yet able to diagnose a mental illness, researchers continue to avidly explore the role of genetics in possible future methods for the diagnosis, treatment, and perhaps even prevention, of mental illness. A goal of a new area of study, pharmacogenetics, is to develop medications to prevent the expression of abnormal genes contributing to mental illnesses (i.e., prevent the passing on of their genetic information).

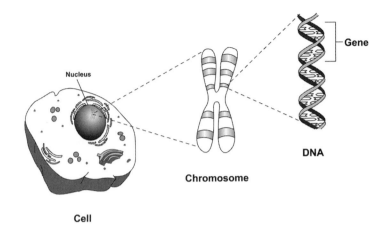

Figure 4.4
The human genome contains the blueprint for all cellular structures and activities for the lifetime of the cell or organism. (Ricochet Productions.)

In her book *Brave New Brain: Conquering Mental Illness in the Age of the Genome*, Nancy C. Andreasen explained: *We often summarize the relative contribution of genes and nongenetic factors by looking at how often identical twins are "concordant" (i.e., manifest the same condition) in comparison with nonidentical twins. This is because identical twins have almost identical genes, while nonidentical twins share only 50% of their genes.* Following is her table showing the relationship of several common mental and physical illnesses:

Concordance Rates in Twins

Types of Illness	Identical Twins	Nonidentical Twins
Autism	60%	5%
Schizophrenia, Bipolar Disorder, Coronary Artery Disease	40%	10%
Depression	50%	15%
Breast Cancer	30%	10%

ENVIRONMENTAL INFLUENCES

As with many physical illnesses, mental illness cannot be blamed purely on biochemical imbalances or on genetics. Environmental factors also play an important role. A person may inherit a genetic predisposition for cardiovascular disease, but smoking, eating high-cholesterol foods, and engaging in too little exercise greatly increases the risk. So it is with mental illness. An individual may be genetically predisposed to biochemical abnormalities that cause depression, for example, but certain types of depression are more likely to manifest following a major emotional trauma. Researchers believe that Huntington's disease is the only mental illness whose causation is almost totally genetic; the rest appear to be multifactorial. Schizophrenia, they believe, is caused partially by genetic influences and partially by environmental influences, and anxiety and mood disorders appear to be more heavily influenced by environmental factors, such as stress or emotional trauma.

IMPORTANCE OF COORDINATING SCIENTIFIC INVESTIGATION

The biopsychosocial model, often studied by behavioral scientists, identifies three components influencing behavior: biological, psychological, and social (environmental). In depression, the biological component may involve genetic predisposition to, or actual imbalances in, brain chemistry; the psychological component may involve negative thoughts or attitudes; and the social component may involve, for example, an abusive relationship. This model has proven to be helpful for research into and treatment of certain mental illnesses. Nancy C. Andreasen, the Andrew H. Woods Chair of Psychiatry at the University of Iowa College of Medicine, Iowa City, wrote of mental illness in *Brave New Brain*: ". . . 'nothing is ever one thing.' If scientists fail to recognize the complexity of causes, they will never find all of them, and perhaps none of them."

Controversies and Issues Surrounding Mental Illness

CHAPTER 5

Validity of the Biomedical Model of Mental Illness: Does Mental Illness Exist?

The Lingering Myth of Mental Illness

Does the concept of mental illness even make sense? It's been almost 30 years now since Thomas Szasz (1960) claimed it does not. . . . Twenty-eight years have passed, yet there has been no real progress in resolving this fundamental debate— whether mental illness truly exists. Of course, to most investigators, mental illness and the various disorders are clearly a reality. As one writer noted: "If schizophrenia is a myth, it is a myth with a strong genetic component!" . . . Perhaps one reason for the continuing debate is the failure of the various interested parties—medicine, psychology, biology . . . to recognize the limitations of their respective domains.

David L. Gilles-Thomas, Lecture Notes, "Mental Illness and Mouse Traps" *(Reprinted by permission of David L. Gilles, Ph.D., website: http://ub-counseling.buffalo.edu/Abpsy/)*

The Western biomedical model of mental illness described in the first section of this book firmly espouses the premise that mental illnesses do, in fact, exist. Modern medical treatment of mental illness, including psychiatric treatment, is therefore based on that premise. However, not all professionals involved in the field of psychiatry agree with the biomedical model, and some even deny the very existence of mental illness. Antipsychiatry movements have existed from the beginnings of psychiatry in the early nineteenth century and have competed ever since with mainstream psychiatry for influence over the treatment of the mentally ill. Members of antipsychiatry movements have variously included psychiatrists, psychologists, neurologists, religious groups, and even mental health care consumers—traditionally called "patients" by mainstream medicine—all seeking to give those diagnosed as being mentally ill a voice and political and legal rights. The practice of forced institutionalization and the horrific treatment of individuals locked in those institutions during the late nineteenth and much of the twentieth centuries sparked increased antipsychiatry activism that continues to this day.

OPPOSITION TO MAINSTREAM PSYCHIATRY

Antipsychiatry

The term "antipsychiatry" was coined in 1967 by the South African psychiatrist David Cooper (1931–1986). It loosely applies to several different philosophies that became prominent in the 1960s, all of which are highly critical of how mental illnesses are diagnosed and treated. Several psychiatrists are considered founders of the antipsychiatry movement, among them Cooper and Ronald David Laing (1927–1989). Cooper was instrumental in establishing the Philadelphia Association in the United Kingdom in 1965, a charitable organization concerned with "the understanding and relief of mental suffering" whose work was based on "a critical engagement with philosophical and psychoanalytical ideas, and a constant questioning of the way society defines mental health and mental illness."

Laing, a Scottish psychiatrist whose views on mental illness were heavily influenced by existential philosophy, did not deny the existence of mental illness or the need for treatment. However, although he rejected the application of the term "antipsychiatry" to his ideas, his opinions were radically different from those of most of his contemporaries and of most twenty-first-century mainstream psychiatrists. In 1960, he presented his opinion that patients classified as mentally ill were simply displaying a "sane response to a mad society." He argued that psychotic episodes are caused by situations in which an individual experiences extreme stress and duress due to inability to conform to conflicting expectations of society and, particularly, family. He saw the confused speech accompanying psychotic states as the individual's attempt to communicate concerns about those stressors, particularly when such communication is unacceptable or not allowed. To Laing, a psychotic episode is a therapeutic and transforming expression of emotional anguish to be valued as a cathartic exercise rather than viewed as a period of insanity. He likened it to a shaman's inward journey—a potentially valuable experience that could help the individual to gain insight and wisdom and therefore to improve his or her life, and he disagreed with the general belief that so-called mental illness is of no fundamental value to the individual. He was also a strong critic of the mainstream method of psychiatric diagnosis, and maintained that it contradicts normal medical procedures in which, in most cases, tests are performed, based upon whose results a diagnosis is made. In contrast, diagnoses of mental illnesses are based on observed behavior and conduct, and only then, if at all, are tests performed.

Many critics of modern psychiatry contend that the cause of mental illness is not biological and that because all human experience is biologically based, no behavioral pattern can be labeled an illness. Some religious groups, such as the Church of Scientology and several fundamentalist Christian organizations, view mental illnesses as spiritual problems and are strongly critical of psychiatry, declaring the profession to be spiritually harmful. Most antipsychiatry proponents agree with the "labeling theory," which contends that labeling an individual as mentally ill not only stigmatizes that individual but encourages or produces the very behavior deemed by psychiatry to be disturbing.

Szasz's Philosophy

Myth of mental illness: Mental illness is a metaphor (metaphorical disease). The word "disease" denotes a demonstrable biological process that affects the bodies of living organisms (plants, animals, and humans). The term "mental illness" refers to the undesirable thoughts, feelings, and behaviors of persons. Classifying thoughts, feelings, and behaviors as diseases is a logical and semantic error, like classifying the whale as a fish. As the whale is not a fish, mental illness is not a disease. Individuals with brain diseases (bad brains) or kidney diseases (bad kidneys) are literally sick. Individuals with mental diseases (bad behaviors), like societies with economic diseases (bad fiscal policies), are metaphorically sick. The classification of (mis)behavior as illness provides an ideological justification for state-sponsored social control as medical treatment.

Thomas Szasz, *Summary Statement and Manifesto, Point 1*
(Reprinted with permission from Dr. T. Szasz and www.szasz.com)

Although he is not an antipsychiatrist, Thomas Szasz (1920–), professor of psychiatry emeritus at the State University of New York's Health Science Center in Syracuse, New York, and an adjunct scholar at the Cato Institute in Washington, D.C., is an outspoken critic of the biomedical model of mental illness. In 1961, he published *The Myth of Mental Illness* to worldwide fame and controversy, and the "myth of mental illness" later became a frequent mantra for those in the antipsychiatry movement.

Among his many arguments is that there is no such thing as mental illness in any culture or in any form because the concept of mental illness is based on flawed methodology and fundamental mistakes. He criticizes all scientific attempts to define mental illness as being nothing but pseudo-science, comparable to astrology or alchemy. Mental illnesses, Szasz argues, are nothing but undesirable thoughts, feelings, and behaviors. He holds that the mind (the mental) is not properly part of the body and, therefore, that the mental is nonphysical because it refers to some of the activities of the brain (which is physical), but not to the brain itself. The brain may develop a disease, such as a tumor or cancer, but the mind cannot. He declares that the proper use of the word "disease" always refers to bodily disease, so that the mind cannot be diseased or ill. From this perspective, those diagnosed as being mentally ill are only metaphorically ill, just as a diseased society can only metaphorically be diseased.

Relativist Perspective   The basic premise of those who support the relativist perspective is that statements pertaining to mental illness can be true in some cultures and false in others. One related premise is that reality is constructed by the mind and is therefore relative to an individual's framework, which includes one's history, culture, family, and individual circumstances. Another related premise is that truth itself is constructed by the mind and, as such, is different for each individual, relative to his or her framework. Therefore, so-called psychiatrically or mentally ill individuals simply have belief systems that differ from those generally held by the culture in which they live. These individuals may generally agree with their culture's idea of truth or reality, but their personal perceptions of reality or truth, and therefore their own reality or truth, differ from that of their cultural environment. People are therefore considered mentally ill only when someone else, or even they themselves, consider their thoughts, emotions, or behavior to be contrary to what their culture or society expects or deems acceptable.

SCIENCE OR NOT?

Szasz and many others who criticize the biomedical model of psychiatry contend that diagnoses based on the biomedical model are nonscientific because there are no scientific tests or objective criteria for mental illness or health. They purport that such diagnoses are based on nonfalsifiable hypotheses that cannot be tested without resorting to virtually unthinkable, inhumane human experiments. In the words of the eminent Austrian-born scientist and social and political philosopher Sir Karl Popper (1902–1994), "if it isn't falsifiable, it isn't empirically testable—and if it is not empirically testable, it is not science at all."

Due to increasing scientific advances, such as brain imaging, drug effectiveness, and genetic investigations, certain of Szasz's arguments have lost a considerable amount of their credibility. Despite this, many critics of mainstream psychiatry argue that even though brain imaging shows certain neuronal changes in some patients with some mental illnesses, there is no concrete evidence as to whether those changes are the cause or the result of the illness. It is known that emotional traumas that are greater than an individual's ability to cope with them can cause long-lasting changes in brain chemistry, as can patterns of learned behavior. And although certain drugs eliminate the symptoms of many mental illnesses, leading to the biomedical hypothesis that imbalances in the levels of certain neurotransmitters may cause the disorder, there again is no clear evidence as to whether those imbalances are the cause or the result of the disorder, and no laboratory test can yet measure brain chemical levels precisely.

From a hereditary perspective, certain mental illnesses seem to run in families, and certain genetic mutations appear to correlate with some mental illnesses. However, there is no definitive evidence that any mental illness, apart from Hodgkin's disease, has genetic roots. Because science cannot prove biological or genetic causes of mental illnesses and has not yet found a cure for any of them, Szasz and others are adamant that psychiatry based on the biomedical model is serously flawed science.

Szasz's viewpoints created significant, heated, and ongoing debates over many issues, including but certainly not limited to the following:

1. Is or is not the mind part of the body? As seen in Chapter 1, many psychiatrists argue that brain and mind are two parts of the same whole.
2. When empirical (observable) evidence shows that certain drugs and treatment modalities alleviate symptoms associated with certain mental illnesses, can mainstream psychiatry be accused of being a pseudoscience simply because there are as yet no definitive tests or falsifiable hypotheses to confirm a diagnosis?
3. To be classified as a disease, must a condition be associated with the physical body only?

Can Mental Illnesses Be Objectively Diagnosed and Classified?

First, if Szasz's insistence that that there is no such thing as mental illness is accurate, then it is impossible to create legitimate diagnostic or classification methods under the biomedical model. Second, as already noted, even antipsychiatrists who do admit that mental illnesses exist have serious concerns that societal values, morals, and ethics too frequently affect diagnosis and classification. Two significant issues in this realm are the following: What conditions should be classified as mental illnesses rather than as part of the range of normal behavior? Once those conditions are agreed upon, how can they be subclassified into different groups?

When a certain behavior is classified in some cultures as a mental illness but in others is considered to be normal or even expected, can that behavior genuinely be classified as a mental illness based on science? Or is such a classification only based on issues of cultural morals and values, of appropriate or inappropriate actions, and of acceptable or unacceptable behavior? Take suicide, for example. In Western culture, serious contemplation of suicide and the act itself is considered to be caused primarily by a mental disorder—bipolar disorder, schizophrenia, depression, or anxiety. That was not always the case. In his book *Why Suicide?* the psychologist Eustace Chesser noted that in Celtic culture, those who committed suicide before illness or the aging process took away their "powers" went to heaven, whereas those who did not went to hell—a concept diametrically opposed to Christian values. Another culture in which suicide is socially acceptable is that of Japan, where, on a personal level, it is considered honorable to commit hara-kiri after seriously "losing face" or failing. On a national level, and for a greater cause, Japanese kamikaze pilots during World War II were ordered to fly their aircraft into U.S. naval vessels, and they did so willingly. Finally, the actions of the Muslim Al Qaeda operatives in the September 11, 2001, terrorist attacks in the United States were suicide missions by individuals who considered themselves—and were considered by other members of their organization— to be martyrs who had earned a place in heaven, as were those of the suicide bombers during the Iraq war that began in 2003. Even in Western culture, people who sacrifice their lives to save another, whether in war or in a rescue mission, are considered heroes. Yet individuals who take their own lives because they feel can no longer cope with a personal situation—in other words, those who have a "selfish" motive—are considered mentally ill. Is, then, the diagnosis of mental illness that is attached to most suicidal tendencies based on objective diagnostic criteria or on moral or ethical issues?

And take homosexuality, the perception of which varies with cultural biases, as another example. When the DSM-II was published in 1968, homosexuality was listed as a psychiatric disease and classified as one of the "sexual deviations." However, in 1973, the American Psychiatric Association (APA) voted to remove homosexuality from the DSM and has ever since eliminated it from subsequent versions. Critics of the biomedical model use this example to support their argument that diagnoses of mental illnesses can be seriously influenced by moralistic and value judgments rather than being solidly based on scientific evidence.

Mental illnesses are classified according to symptoms that cannot definitively be linked to a cause, whereas most medical symptoms can be attributed to a cause. Dr. Jerrold S. Maxmen wrote in his 1985 book *The New Psychiatry*: "It is generally unrecognized that psychiatrists are the *only* medical specialists who treat disorders that, by definition, have no definitively known causes or cures. . . . A diagnosis should indicate the cause of a mental disorder, but . . . since the etiologies of most mental disorders are unknown, current diagnostic systems can't reflect them."

The Fight against Coercive Psychiatry

Perhaps the strongest thread uniting Szasz and his followers with the proponents of antipsychiatry is their common opposition to legalized coercive psychiatry in any form, particularly to forced drug, electroconvulsive, or surgical treatments, as well as to institutionalization, with its dehumanizing and often damaging and deadly results. While many antipsychiatry proponents do not deny that psychiatric patients may be mentally ill, they nevertheless vehemently oppose involuntary treatment from a civil liberties perspective.

Then there is the argument that because diagnoses cannot be confirmed scientifically, they can easily be used as a means of social and political control, such as occurred during the Nazi era when they were used as a method of racial and political cleansing, and during more recent times to subdue political dissidents in Russia, China, and other countries.

The following quote is from personal e-mail communication with Professor Jeffrey A. Schaler, Department of Justice, Law and Society, School of Public Affairs, American University, Washington, D.C. Schaler is also the owner and producer of The Thomas S. Szasz Cybercenter for Liberty and Responsibility Web site.

Just please don't call Szasz (or me) an "antipsychiatrist!" We believe in psychiatry between consenting adults. We're not for banning mood-changing drugs. We think people should be able to put whatever drug they want into their bodies just as they should be able to put whatever ideas they want into their minds. You see, people who consider themselves "antipsychiatrists" are opposed to allowing these drugs on the free market. We are completely opposed to their position. We also believe that people should be free to see a psychiatrist or any other "mental health professional" if they want to, regardless of whether they consider mental illness to exist or not—the point is, NO COERCION.

Reprinted with permission from J. A. Schaler and www.szasz.com

Citizens Commission on Human Rights

In 1969, Szasz and the Church of Scientology cofounded the Citizens Commission on Human Rights (CCHR), a highly effective activist organization that by 2005 had 133 chapters in thirty-four countries fighting crimes against human rights committed by the mental health industry in the name of mental health. The following information appears on the CCHR Web site:

- Between 1950 and 1964, more people died in U.S. psychiatric hospitals than were killed in the Revolutionary War, the War of 1812, the Mexican War, the Civil War, the Spanish-American War, World Wars I and II, the Korean War, the Vietnam War and the Persian Gulf War combined. In fact, between 1950 and 1990, the total number of psychiatric inpatient deaths exceeded the cumulative number of war casualties by at least 70%.
- Between 1998 and 1999, 150 people died from restraint procedures in psychiatric facilities in the United States. Thirteen of these deaths over a 2-year period were of teenagers and children placed under psychiatric "care."

Exposure of such deaths, almost always called "unfortunate accidents" or blamed on natural causes, resulted in a U.S. regulation passed in 1999 prohibiting physical and chemical restraint as disciplinary or coercive measures against the mentally ill. The regulation also enforced a mandatory reporting system for all psychiatric facilities by denying funds to any institution ignoring the regulation. This regulation did not stop some institutions from using restraint, particularly on children. According to CCHR, 17-year-old Charles Chase Moody died while restrained in a behavioral treatment center in Mason County, Texas, on October 14, 2002, the fifth death in that chain of facilities since 1998.

Some who challenge coercive psychiatry may not disagree that it is sometimes necessary to treat or to hospitalize some extremely mentally ill individuals. Their primary concern is that society is far too quick to use pharmaceuticals or hospitalization for individuals who have only minor disorders or who are arbitrarily accused of being a danger to themselves or others, and that in many other instances individuals are forcibly and unnecessarily drugged or institutionalized for years.

Achievements

Although organizations against mainstream psychiatry are highly criticized by many in the medical and psychiatric communities, they have accomplished thousands of liberating and protective acts and activities, both nationally and internationally. Such antipsychiatry movements had gained considerable respect by the 1970s, which prompted laws against some of the worst psychiatric abuses. In 1999, for instance, the United States Supreme Court enacted a law against unnecessary confinement of disabled individuals, including confinement of mentally disabled in institutions. Subsequent to the legislation, however, forty-two states legalized alternative treatment methods by allowing court-ordered involuntary psychiatric drug treatment for mentally ill outpatients.

The effort toward community care for the mentally ill can be attributed in part to efforts from antipsychiatry and similar organizations. In 2002, President George W. Bush ordered the establishment of the President's New Freedom Commission on Mental Health, which states, "The mission of the Commission shall be to conduct a comprehensive study of the United States mental health service delivery system, including public and private sector providers, and to advise the President on methods of improving the system. The Commission's goal shall be to recommend improvements to enable adults with serious mental illness and children with serious emotional disturbances to live, work, learn, and participate fully in their communities."

In their ongoing efforts, CCHR appeared before the commission in Los Angeles, California, on 13 November 2003 and presented a report titled "The Silent Death of America's Children," in which they exposed the history of dozens of children who died during the 1990s and early 2000s as a result of psychiatric treatment involving psychotropic medication and restraint.

CCHR and other organizations opposing mainstream psychiatry, such as the Psychiatric Survivors Movement, MindFreedom International, the International Center for the Study of Psychiatry and Psychology, and the United States Libertarian Party, have helped those diagnosed as mentally ill obtain legal rights, particularly in the realm of unjustified and lengthy institutionalization, restraint, and forced drug treatment. They have also spurred many active survivor/consumer groups consisting of individuals who experienced devastating consequences of mainstream perspectives toward mental illnesses, such as stigmatization, institutionalization, broken relationships, and loss of employment and self-esteem. Such groups encourage an individual vision of recovery and an attitude of wellness, independence, self-determination, and control over one's own life, rather than seeing oneself as a passive victim of chemical imbalances destined to perpetual illness and dependency on psychiatry. They have developed peer and community self-help support services as alternatives that can be used instead of, or in conjunction, with traditional mental health services.

The following information is posted on the Citizens Commission on Human Rights International Web site in the section titled "Involuntary Commitment":

In 1969, Hungarian refugee Victor Gyory was committed to Haverford State Hospital in Philadelphia, stripped naked, held in isolation against his will and forced to undergo electroshock. He was refused the right to an attorney and denied the right to refuse treatment. CCHR obtained the aid of Hungarian-born Dr. Thomas Szasz, who discovered that Gyory had been diagnosed as "schizophrenic with paranoid tendencies" for one simple reason—his inability to speak English. Chief counsel for CCHR prepared to take Gyory's case to court to test the constitutionality of Pennsylvania's law, at which point the hospital director discharged Gyory.

CHAPTER 6

Political Acts and Legal Issues: Protection or Discrimination?

> Separation of Psychiatry and the State: If we recognize that "mental illness" is a metaphor for disapproved thoughts, feelings, and behaviors, we are compelled to recognize as well that the primary function of Psychiatry is to control thought, mood, and behavior. Hence, like Church and State, Psychiatry and the State ought to be separated by a "wall." At the same time, the State ought not to interfere with mental health practices between consenting adults. The role of psychiatrists and mental health experts with regard to law, the school system, and other organizations ought to be similar to the role of clergymen in those situations."
>
> Thomas Szasz, *Summary Statement and Manifesto, Point 2*
> *(Reprinted with permission from Dr. T. Szasz and www.szasz.com)*

Federal and state laws concerning constitutional rights of people diagnosed with mental illness are surrounded by heated debate on all levels—from governments, to law-enforcement agencies and officials, to providers of mental health services, to insurance companies, to researchers, and to mental health consumers, their family members, and their advocates. Three particularly contentions issues are involuntary commitment and outpatient treatment, the insanity defense, and privacy versus disclosure.

INVOLUNTARY COMMITMENT

Involuntary commitment is a complex process by which certain individuals diagnosed with a mental illness can be placed in a psychiatric institution or hospital unit or treated on an outpatient basis without their informed consent. Each state has its own laws, and although they may differ somewhat, they generally require that a court of law find the individual to be a potential danger to self or others. The commitment process must follow rigid criteria and can only be initiated by someone with firsthand knowledge of the individual in question.

In a typical emergency commitment scenario, regardless of illness severity, a petition or emergency commitment order is issued by a magistrate, valid for up to 72 hours, asserting that the individual is mentally ill and requires immediate commitment to protect that person or others from physical harm. Once the individual is in police custody, he or she must be examined by a physician or psychologist within a designated time period— for example, 24 hours. If the examiner determines the need for involuntary treatment, the court orders hospitalization. Once committed, the individual must be examined a second time, within another designated time period—often 12 hours—by another psychiatrist. Within 24 hours, a copy of the petition must be given to the individual's attorney, parent, or guardian. Within 72 hours, the individual, who is entitled to legal representation or to be provided with a public defender, must appear before a judge, who has authority to extend the order. The hospitalized individual is assured certain rights, such as contact with people outside the facility, and must be reevaluated periodically.

Evolution of Involuntary Commitment Laws

The U.S. Declaration of Independence and Constitution incorporated into the fundamental laws of the nation three basic principles defined by Aristotle in the fourth century BC:

1. Informed consent: a process by which an individual embarks on an endeavor willingly, knowingly, and rationally, and that legally protects that individual from force or coercion. Informed consent is pertinent to events such as marriage, medical treatment, entering into a contract, and confessing to law enforcement officials.
2. Police power: the power of government to protect its citizens from danger and harm.
3. *Parens patriae*: Latin for "parent of the nation," referring to the government's responsibility to assist the needy who have no other means of assistance.

These principles are the fundamental center of debate and conflict surrounding involuntary treatment of the mentally ill. Opponents of involuntary treatment argue that it violates an individual's constitutional civil rights and liberties because the individual is denied the right to informed consent. Proponents argue in favor of the government's constitutional power and responsibility.

Why Involuntary Commitment Laws?   In the sixteenth century, involuntary civil commitment became a formalized means for government to remove and isolate "undesirables" from communities. No distinction was made between the homeless, vagrants, drunkards, criminals, or the mentally ill. In Paris, France, peasants driven from their farms, impoverished scholars, the unemployed, and the physically and mentally ill who were homeless were incarcerated and used as forced labor. In England, the poor and homeless mentally ill were confined to what were commonly called poorhouses under harsh and often fatal living conditions. All through the seventeenth century, the mentally ill were incarcerated with criminals, social deviants, and the homeless disabled.

In early colonial America, there was no governmental help for those unable to support themselves, and there were few jails and prisons. The mentally ill were cared for by family members—when they had them, and if those members wanted them. Large groups of indigents, mentally ill, and others ostracized by communities wandered from town to town. As prisons were built, many of these drifters, including the mentally ill, were simply locked up with criminals. Only with the minor reform measures and the building of one mental asylum during the mid-1700s did the government and society begin taking some responsibility for the mentally ill. Even by the mid-1800s, most mentally ill people were still locked in jails and almshouses under appalling, dehumanizing conditions.

Boston schoolteacher Dorothea Lynde Dix (1802–1887), horrified by what she saw after going to a prison to teach Sunday school, started a social movement that triggered the establishment of many more asylums intended to provide compassionate care for the mentally ill. Despite the good intentions, asylums eventually became places of imprisonment and abuse. Laws governing involuntary commitment were inadequate, at best, and commitment again became a method of removing "undesirables" from families and communities: parents committed difficult children; husbands committed difficult wives. One such wife was Elizabeth Parsons Ware Packard (1816–1897) whose husband, the Rev. Theophilus Packard, took advantage of a state regulation that made it much easier for a husband to commit his wife than it was to accomplish any other form of commitment. After her release, Mrs. Packard helped expose her illegal commitment and that of many others. Her passionate campaign resulted in much-needed legislation intended to provide greater protection for the mentally ill.

Reformation: A Long Haul   Because the mentally ill have traditionally been viewed with fear, contempt, and misunderstanding, protecting their civil liberties has been a long, hard battle. As late as the 1970s, when the commitment process was handed over to the courts, involuntary commitment without due legal process was a reality. All it took was for a family member or physician to call the medical examiner, who could then take the individual to a psychiatric hospital. People were often kept for years, decades, or even life under false accusations, often in inhumane, abusive, and neglectful conditions, with no right to appeal and no possibility of release. After World War II, due to the huge influx of patients and accompanying staff shortages, mental institutions became fearful places that were referred to as snake pits. On any given day in the early 1950s, close to 600,000 individuals were in institutions, deprived of all legal rights, and potentially subjected to forced medical procedures and experiments, forced labor, isolation, brutal physical restraint, and drug and electroconvulsive therapy (ECT), as well as the possibility of being denied interaction with family or friends. Horror stories arose of perfectly sane people being completely trapped.

Following a report released in 1960 by the Joint Commission on Mental Illness and Health titled *Action for Mental Health*, awareness of these conditions increased. Politicians and the public alike acknowledged that people with mental illnesses have civil rights, which should be protected as fiercely as the civil rights of the general population. Considerable pressure developed to revamp the state hospital system. Community mental health care was hailed as a more humane and beneficial form of treatment, and in 1963, President John F. Kennedy signed the Community Mental Health Centers Act, which provided for a range of services outside the hospital setting. However, critics noted that there was little or no provision at the community level for chronically psychotic patients who required continuous care.

One of the most important pieces of legislation governing involuntary commitment was California's 1967 Lanterman-Petris-Short (LPS) Act, which defined stringent criteria that must be met for court-ordered commitment. Some form of this act was eventually adopted by almost every state, with the primary purpose of such laws being to prevent inappropriate and indefinite commitment. Once again, although intentions were good, the major problem became—and remains—how to help people who clearly need treatment but do not meet the stringent criteria.

Federal Involvement   The first time the U.S. Supreme Court ruled on a matter involving individual civil liberties was in connection with the desegregation of schools in the mid-1950s. Many more lawsuits followed, as well as subsequent laws concerning other civil rights issues, including rights to privacy and the Miranda rights. Not until 1972, however, did the Court make its first significant decision concerning the civil rights of the mentally ill. In *O'Connor v. Donaldson*, a relatively simple ruling stated that individuals could not be civilly committed against their will strictly on the grounds of being mentally ill as long as they competently understood and accepted their condition and could survive safely by themselves or with assistance from others. The Court maintained that people with a mental illness should be treated no differently than people with a physical illness as long as they pose no danger to themselves or to someone else. Virtually every state adopted the "danger to self or others" standard to protect against flagrant and irresponsible use of involuntary commitment. Federal community mental health centers (CMHCs) were developed, mandated by Congressional law in 1975 to provide comprehensive outpatient care. Some advocates for the mentally ill even spearheaded efforts to close all mental institutions in the name of civil liberty.

Effects of Deinstitutionalization   The 1970s ushered in the era known as deinstitutionalization, initiated by a complicated combination of civil rights advocacy, reduced governmental funding for state hospitals, development of CMHCs, and the introduction of psychotropic medications. Hundreds of thousands of patients were released from mental hospitals. Many were capable of living independently under CMHC care or with help from friends or family. Many difficult cases, including thousands diagnosed as severely and persistently mentally ill (SPMI), needed consistent monitoring and supervision, could not supervise their own medication regimen, and became helpless, homeless, and vulnerable to violence and lived in filthy conditions. Some committed acts of violence due to their psychotic condition and were incarcerated. The laws that protected against inappropriate hospitalization became a double-edged sword, endangering those who required care the most.

In 1977, President Jimmy Carter helped establish the President's Commission on Mental Health, designed to review community mental health needs and make recommendations. This commission found many deinstitutionalized SPMI individuals were at high risk of returning to a hospital, in part because they lacked sufficient community assistance. A new group of mentally ill had developed, known as "revolving-door" patients, who were temporarily hospitalized, improved due to supervised care, were released, and deteriorated again. In 1980, the Mental Health Systems Act was passed, outlining a new national program, but the act was abolished by

President Ronald Reagan as soon as he took office when he declared that
federal funds must be cut. Federal funding for CMHCs were scaled back,
and state and local governments bore the brunt of public mental health
costs. Either unable or unwilling to provide funds, states continued to close
psychiatric hospitals. The number of homeless mentally ill grew, as did the
number arrested and imprisoned. Estimates of the total number of homeless mentally ill in California alone in 1980 ranged from 20,000 to 35,000.

Easing Requirements for Involuntary Treatment   By the close of the
twentieth century, the pendulum was swinging the other way, with laws
being passed to make it easier to have someone treated involuntarily.

Kendra's Law   New York State was the first to challenge the stringent involuntary commitment laws following the death in January 1999 of Kendra
Webdale, a young woman awaiting her train in a New York subway station.
Andrew Goldstein, a 29-year-old man diagnosed with delusional paranoid
schizophrenia who was not taking medication, pushed her into the path of an
oncoming train. The state passed a law, commonly known as Kendra's Law,
that established court procedures to force certain people to receive assisted
outpatient treatment (AOT) or, upon noncompliance with the order, to be
admitted to an inpatient facility. AOT is a mandated, intensive, community-
based treatment for the most severely mentally ill that continues until the individual is deemed well enough and sufficiently responsible enough to manage
his or her own treatment regimen. Although surrounded by controversy and
challenged as unconstitutional, the law was still in effect in 2006.

Kendra's Law and the Failure of the System   In 2000, Goldstein was
sentenced to the maximum of 25 years to life in prison for Webdale's
death. It should be noted, however, that Goldstein never refused treatment. In fact, in the 2 years prior to the incident, he had unsuccessfully
sought help at various hospital emergency rooms for his illness. He was
denied treatment thirteen times. His advocates accuse the public system—
which is required to offer state-financed housing, clinic visits, and an
intensive case manager—of failing in all respects. In an article titled
"Incarceration Is Not a Solution to Mental Illness" on the Prison Policy
Initiative Web site, Peter Wagner wrote, "Kendra's law doesn't provide
for more services, just more repression, and targets all of the mentally ill,
not merely those prone to violence."

Laura's Law   In spite of opposition from civil libertarians and mental
health consumers, many other states followed New York's lead, making

involuntary commitment and AOT easier to obtain. Although it relaxed AOT laws much later than most states, California passed a bill in 2003 known as Laura's Law, so named for 19-year-old Laura Wilcox, one of three people shot to death at a Nevada City public mental health clinic in January 2001 by Scott Harlan Thorpe, an enraged 41-year-old suffering from delusional paranoia. He was convinced the FBI was trying to poison his food and refused his family's attempts to get him into treatment. California's requirements for AOT intervention include dangerousness, hospitalization twice in the preceding 3 years or violence in the preceding 4 years, likelihood of not being able to live alone safely and without supervision, and likelihood to become ill enough without AOT to require inpatient treatment.

Controversies Surrounding Involuntary Commitment

What becomes of SPMI individuals unable to care for themselves in the community? Is treatment without the individual's informed consent beneficial therapy or a restraint technique? Should informed consent always be required, even when the individual is unaware of his or her illness or is unable to maintain his or her own treatment regimen? Is it ever appropriate to use police power or *parens patriae* to deprive someone diagnosed as SPMI of their civil liberties on the grounds that they *might* be a danger to self or others? Are SPMI individuals more dangerous than the general population?

Opponents' Arguments

Abolition of involuntary mental hospitalization: Involuntary mental hospitalization is imprisonment under the guise of treatment; it is a covert form of social control that subverts the rule of law. No one ought to be deprived of liberty except for a criminal offense, after a trial by jury guided by legal rules of evidence. No one ought to be detained against his will in a building called "hospital," or in any other medical institution, or on the basis of expert opinion. Medicine ought to be clearly distinguished and separated from penology, treatment from punishment, the hospital from the prison. No person ought to be detained involuntarily for a purpose other than punishment or in an institution other than one formally defined as a part of the state's criminal justice system.

Thomas Szasz, *Summary Statement and Manifesto, Point 4*
(Reprinted with permission from Dr. T. Szasz and www.szasz.com)

As noted, a major criticism of involuntary commitment concerns civil liberty and constitutional issues. Opponents of commitment dispute the constitutionality of laws that allow an individual, in any situation, to be deprived of liberty, either by imprisonment, hospitalization, or forced treatment, solely on the grounds that—in the opinion of one or more psychiatrists or other so-called experts—that individual has the *potential* or is *perceived* to be a possible danger to self or others and *might* commit a crime. Some argue that involuntary commitment and treatment laws are simply a means of controlling certain individuals or groups determined by governmental and other authorities, including mental health experts or families, as dissident, difficult to control, or problematic. Such laws clearly create a class of people who can be arrested briefly for having committed no crime and then subsequently "detained" (some call it imprisoned) in a treatment facility under the guise of protective custody. In contrast, an individual *not* classified as mentally ill cannot legally be detained on similar grounds. Even the civil liberties of criminals are protected by due legal process: individuals can only be detained *after* committing a crime and sentenced to imprisonment *after* being found guilty in court. This right is denied to anyone classified as mentally ill. Dr. Jeffrey Schaler, a psychologist and an adjunct professor at American University's School of Public Affairs in Washington, D.C., commented on The Szasz Blog Web site: "The U.S. Constitution does not say at the end, 'PS: For mentally healthy people only.'"

Closely associated with the civil liberty issue is the constitutional right of an individual to give informed consent regarding treatment. If an individual is committed involuntarily, that person is then subject to whatever treatment is deemed appropriate by the institution's staff, which may be strong psychotropic medication, restraint, or ECT. Critics point to hundreds of such incidents that surface each year. As a case in point, in 2002, after hearing testimony from staff psychiatrists, a personal physician, and others, a court in Minnesota ruled that a civilly committed 48-year-old woman diagnosed with paranoid schizophrenia, depression, anxiety disorder, and disorders not otherwise specified (NOS), could be treated with fifteen sessions of ECT per week for 5 weeks, followed by regular maintenance therapy "at an unspecified duration for the remainder of the commitment." The court concluded that there was sufficient evidence that the patient was incompetent to either give or withhold consent to treatment, and that the benefits of treatment outweighed the risks and justified "intrusion into her privacy as needed to conduct the electroconvulsive therapy without Respondent's informed consent." Even in states such as Michigan in which ECT without the patient's informed consent is illegal, courts still often permit it.

Another question often argued is whether SPMI individuals are more likely to be of danger to self or others than members of the general population. One study followed 20,000 people for 18 months after hospitalization, treatment, and release. During that 18-month period, only thirty-three were arrested for violent crimes, almost all of whom had a criminal record prior to hospitalization. Those who had no previous criminal record were less likely to be arrested than members of the general population. On the other hand, according to a 2003 briefing paper posted on the Treatment and Advocacy Center Web site, other studies show that those who remain untreated are more dangerous than the general population.

Criticism of Assisted Outpatient Treatment As of June 2004, only Connecticut, Maine, Maryland, Massachusetts, New Jersey, New Mexico, Nevada, and Tennessee had no laws governing outpatient treatment. Arguments made against AOT laws adopted by all other states include the following:

- The structure of these laws intrudes on the individual's constitutional right to make their own treatment decisions.
- Coercive treatment programs require individuals to surrender certain degrees of autonomy and control over their own lives and impacts their sense of dignity.
- Due to the coercive nature of outpatient commitment, people who may otherwise voluntarily seek treatment may avoid the mental health system out of fear of forced treatment or hospitalization.
- Although the patient can legally provide input into his or her AOT plan, that input is minimal because the treatment plan is in place before the patient is consulted.
- Court-ordered treatment increases the stigma surrounding mental illness, giving the public the impression that mentally ill people are different, irresponsible, dangerous, and unable to control their own lives.
- AOT laws require the "least restrictive" form of treatment, which means an individual can opt to be treated voluntarily. However, in an April 15, 2005, article by Michelle Chen on The New Standard Web site, Dennis Feld, a lawyer with Mental Hygiene Legal Services in New York who assists individuals facing AOT, is quoted as saying that even in the 20–30 percent of cases in which an individual does request voluntary treatment, AOT administrators still push the judge for court-ordered treatment, claiming that the individual lacks the necessary judgment to comply voluntarily.
- Although some studies report a high overall success rate of AOT laws, the science behind those reports still lies in question, with claims that there is lack of valid evidence that such laws effectively

improve treatment compliance, increase public safety, or reduce rehospitalization rates.

- A 2000 report by the RAND Corporation, a nonprofit research and analysis group, found slim evidence that AOT is effective and that there is no evidence that shows that a court order is necessary for compliance or has any independent effect on outcomes.
- A researcher employed by the New York State Office of Mental Health (OMH) from 1996 to 2005 found that his efforts to design a study assessing the effects of AOT following implementation of Kendra's Law were thwarted by other OMH officials who demanded final authority over the way the results would be presented. The official claims that the government has yet to appropriately assess the effects of the law.

- The laws impact a disproportionate number of minorities:

  - According to Chen's article, from 1999 to 2004, under Kendra's Law, 42 and 21 percent of all court AOT orders involved Blacks and Hispanics, respectively, whereas Blacks and Hispanics constituted only 16 and 15 percent, respectively, of the state's population. The 2003 statewide mental health patient survey also indicated that of all adult SPMI individuals, approximately 24 percent were Blacks and 17 percent Hispanics.

- Well-financed and well-administered community mental health support services provide easier access and a better alternative, reducing emotional trauma, stigma, violation of legal rights, and the high legal costs of forced treatment.
- AOT laws wrongly judge anyone who has an impaired awareness of their mental illness and who therefore does not seek voluntary treatment as being legally incompetent; however, if that same individual agrees to treatment, he or she is deemed legally competent.
- A review published by doctors Marvin S. Swartz and Jeffrey W. Swanson in the *Canadian Journal of Psychiatry* found that outpatient commitment (OPC) is only effective if combined with frequent and comprehensive community services. The system focuses and relies on coercive treatment rather than on comparably effective community services geared toward voluntary treatment.

  - Following the enactment of Kendra's Law, New York State funded the AOT program to the tune of $157 million while continuing to slash billions of dollars from the general community mental health budget. In the words of one mental health consumer quoted in Chen's article: "[If] I seek treatment voluntarily, I'm denied services, but if I'm willing to forfeit all of my constitutional rights, I can get all the treatment I want."

Proponents' Arguments

To proponents of Kendra's law, what is unacceptable is that the state should be barred from imposing what they view as treatment in order to serve the public interest.

Michelle Chen, "Law to Force Mental Illness Treatment
Raises Ire of Civil Libertarians"

Proponents of involuntary treatment raise a myriad of issues to support their point of view. One major argument is the dramatic increase in incarceration of individuals diagnosed as SPMI since deinstitutionalization (Table 6.1). Advocate Richard Elliott, a psychiatrist at Mercer University School of Medicine in Macon, Georgia, commented in at article by Don Schanche, Jr. in the *Macon Telegraph*: "Nobody was really deinstitutionalized. They were trans-institutionalized to other institutions, like nursing homes or jails. . . . We've sort of gone back to the Dorothea Dix days." The same article quoted psychiatrist E. Fuller Torrey from his 1998 study: "One predictable consequence is that an increasing number of these discharged patients ended up in jail. The three largest de facto psychiatric inpatient facilities in the United States are now the Los Angeles County jail, the Rikers Island jail in New York City and Cook County jail in Chicago." Wagner, too, noted that Rikers Island houses approximately 130,000 inmates over the course of a year, 20 percent of whom are SPMI and 80 percent of whom have a substance abuse problem. Pertinent to this argument is that in 1999, New York eliminated 500 psychiatric inpatient beds yet funded psychiatric wings in two huge new prisons to the tune of $360 million.

Another serious issue is how to effectively treat SPMI individuals who refuse treatment or are unable to supervise their own treatment regimen. According to several studies, individuals who are SPMI often do not know

Table 6.1 **Comparison of the Number of Mentally Ill Patients in New York State Hospitals and Department of Corrections: 1973 and 2000**

Year	State Hospitals	State Department of Corrections
1973	93,000	12,500
2000	5,000	72,000

they are ill, which is the primary reason for nontreatment and treatment noncompliance. Many mental health consumers believe involuntary treatment saved their lives because they were either unaware of their illness or could not make a decision to seek treatment. In many cases, family members consider involuntary hospitalization the only means of preventing a loved one with an SPMI from falling into homelessness or incarceration. Schanche quoted Torrey: "We changed the laws to make it virtually impossible to treat anyone against their will, even if they have no awareness of their illness."

By the early 2000s, those attempting to make involuntary treatment easier were calling for broader definitions of the "danger to self and others" criteria. They also wanted an individual's mental health history permitted in the court's consideration. Critics opposed the latter on the grounds that it is unconstitutional under the right to privacy laws. In 2002, California passed a law containing such a provision, bill AB 1424, which states that the individual's medical records and information from family members, police, and the individual or a representative must be presented as evidence of mental health history. Police could consider information from family members when deciding if the patient should be taken into custody for evaluation and treatment. Furthermore, insurance companies were no longer permitted to use either voluntary or involuntary commitment as a basis for refusal of coverage. Proponents of the law believe it improves the quality of evidence upon which court-ordered treatment is based and is an incentive for the individual in question to choose voluntary commitment and therefore receive medically necessary services, without the risk of being denied insurance payments.

Other arguments put forth by proponents include the following:

- It saves lives by preventing suicide:

  - Most cases of involuntary commitment are due to suicidal tendencies. More than 30,000 Americans commit suicide each year, and more than 90 percent of all suicides are committed by people diagnosed with a mental illness.

- It protects the mentally ill from becoming victims of violence, providing them, instead, with a safe place and a sense of well-being.

  - The rate of violent victimization of individuals with an SPMI is an estimated 3 million annually, eleven times higher than in the general population.
  - Lifetime risk of violent crimes, including sexual assault, against homeless mentally ill women is 97 percent.

- Most acts of violence against mentally ill individuals go unreported, and even when they are, the reports are often ignored.

- It protects the public from violent acts by individuals with severe mental illnesses. Although the rate of violent crimes committed by the SPMI is far lower than in the general population, approximately 5 percent of all homicides are committed by people diagnosed with a mental illness. According to a 1994 Department of Justice report, of the number of people murdered by a family member with untreated mental illness in 1988,

  - 12.3 percent were killed by a spouse
  - 15.8 percent were killed by a parent
  - 25.1 percent were killed by a child
  - 17.3 percent were killed by a sibling

- It reduces homelessness. In contrast to less than 5 percent of the general U.S. population, approximately 20–40 percent of the homeless population suffers from an SPMI.
- It helps the indigent obtain care they may otherwise not be able to afford.
- It helps prevent the "revolving door" syndrome of repeated hospitalization, imprisonment, and homelessness.
- It lowers the overall fiscal costs to the community; incarceration costs more and is less effective than treatment.
- AOT laws give access to the limited services that are available to those who need them most.
- A 5-year study of the effects of Kendra's Law published by the OMH found that as of March 2005, 3,908 individuals received AOT orders. Compared with the 3 years prior to participation in the program, AOT recipients experienced

  - 74 percent reduction in homelessness
  - 77 percent reduction in psychiatric hospitalization
  - 83 percent reduction in arrest
  - 87 percent less incarceration

- An interview with seventy-six AOT recipients found that although half were initially angry or embarrassed by court-ordered treatment, following treatment

  - 75 percent felt it helped them regain control over their lives
  - 81 percent felt it improved their condition

- 90 percent found they were more likely to be responsible in keeping their appointments and taking their medication.

INSANITY DEFENSE

Abolition of the insanity defense: Insanity is a legal concept involving the courtroom determination that a person is not capable of forming conscious intent and, therefore, cannot be held responsible for an otherwise criminal act. The opinions of experts about the "mental state" of defendants ought to be inadmissible in court, exactly as the opinions of experts about the "religious state" of defendants are inadmissible. No one ought to be excused of lawbreaking or any other offense on the basis of so-called expert opinion rendered by psychiatric or mental health experts. Excusing a person of responsibility for an otherwise criminal act on the basis of inability to form conscious intent is an act of legal mercy masquerading as an act of medical science. Being merciful or merciless toward lawbreakers is a moral and legal matter, unrelated to the actual or alleged expertise of medical and mental health professionals.

Thomas Szasz, *Summary Statement and Manifesto, Point 5*
(Reprinted with permission from Dr. T. Szasz and www.szasz.com)

In most states, laws allow a defendant to use the defense of being insane at the time of the crime. Laws differ from state to state and have changed over the years from strict to more lenient to strict once again. This particular defense is used in less than 1 percent of criminal trials, it is successful in only approximately 26 percent of those instances, and in 80 percent of successful cases, defense and prosecution agree prior to the trial that it is an appropriate plea.

Not Guilty by Reason of Insanity

In the legal system, the definition of insanity—which is a legal term only and not a medical definition—differs from the psychiatric definition of mental illness. The insanity test is the basis for courtroom battles pertaining to a plea of not guilty by reason of insanity (NGRI). Simply having a mental disease, disorder, or defect is not sufficient. Being found NGRI does not mean that the defendant is not guilty of the crime but that the defendant is deemed to have been so mentally ill or mentally incompetent at the time of the crime that he or she was either unaware of or unable to appreciate the nature and quality of the wrongfulness of the act or unable to control his or her behavior. The basic principle behind the defense, argued by some to be flawed, is that willful intent is a necessary component of most offenses, but a mentally incompetent person is unable to meet that criterion and therefore should not be punished for his or her crime. The verdict as to whether the defendant is NGRI is entirely up to the jury. To help jurors make that determination, they hear testimony of "expert" witnesses, usually psychiatrists, on behalf of both the prosecution and defense. If found NGRI, the defendant is usually confined for treatment in a psychiatric hospital for the severely mentally ill who have committed a crime. No specific time period is mandated by the court; rather, the institution's authorities determine when and if an individual no longer poses a threat to society, and time spent in the institution is almost always longer than a prison sentence established for that particular crime. Such committed individuals were often held indefinitely, with no legal recourse. Concerns about civil rights for the mentally ill that arose in the 1960s and 1970s resulted in indefinite confinement laws being overturned in many states, along with the enactment of laws requiring periodic evaluation of the committed individual's mental condition and level of danger. Forty-two states adopted these reforms by the mid-1980s. Not until 1992, however, in *Foucha v. Louisiana*, did the U.S.. Supreme Court outlaw indefinite confinement.

Evolution of NGRI Laws

The insanity defense existed in the Greek and Roman judicial systems. In 1581, a treatise in Britain stated "If a madman or a natural fool, or a lunatic in the time of his lunacy do [kill a man], this is no felonious act for they cannot be said to have any understanding will." The first recorded trial in which the insanity defense was used was in 1724. Modern use of the defense stems from the 1843 trial in British courts in which Daniel M'Naughten, a Scottish woodcutter, attempted to murder England's prime minister. Although he failed to do do, he succeeded in murdering the prime minister's secretary. At the juried trial, nine witnesses testified M'Naughten was insane, and he was found "not guilty by reason of insanity." Queen Victoria sent the verdict to the House of Lords for review, and although a panel of judges reversed the verdict, they declared that from thenceforth, a defendant should not be held responsible if unable to distinguish whether his or her actions were wrong when the crime was committed. Their decision became the foundation of the insanity defense in English courts and was adopted by American courts. The M'Naughten rule underwent few changes until the mid–twentieth century. In fact, twenty-five states and the District of Columbia were still using modified versions of the rule in 1998.

Over the years in the United States, modifications were made to the M'Naughten rule, one being the addition of the "irresistible impulse" provision under which an individual may also be legally absolved. The premise underlying this provision is that a person may understand their intended action is wrong yet be unable to control the impulse to commit the crime due to their mental state. In the 1950s, the law was criticized from both the legal and the psychiatric perspectives, with calls for the addition of medical evidence of mental illness to substantiate an insanity plea. As described in a *PBS Frontline* report titled "A Crime of Insanity," a 1954 ruling by the U.S. Court of Appeals in the District of Columbia in *Durham v. United States* introduced a "mental disease or defect" ruling, under which a defendant could not be judged responsible "if his unlawful act was the product of mental disease or mental defect." In 1962, the American Law Institute (ALI) further softened existing laws with what is often called the "substantial capacity test," a provision that "as a result of a mental disease or defect, [the defendant] lacks substantial capacity either to appreciate the criminality of his conduct or to conform his conduct to the requirements of the law." The 1972 Brawner Rule permitted juries rather than psychiatrists to decide whether or not the insanity defense applied in any given case. In 1975, the U.S. Supreme Court ruled in *Ford v. Wainwright* that prisoners legally deemed insane could not be executed.

In 1981, laws were introduced making the NGRI defense more difficult. That year, John Hinckley, Jr. attempted to assassinate President Ronald Reagan and shot four of the president's staff members. Hinckley was clearly delusional and was acquitted by a jury of thirteen counts, including murder, by reason of insanity as defined by the 1962 ALI law. A huge public outcry ensued, and Congress passed twenty-six different pieces of legislation aimed at completely abolishing the insanity defense. This public and political outrage was countered by lawyers and psychiatrists, and a compromise between the opposing parties resulted in the Insanity Defense Reform Act of 1984. While the NGRI defense provision would remain, the 1962 substantial capacity test law was overturned. Federal and many state governments reverted to laws closely resembling the 1843 M'Naughten law. Before the Hinckley acquittal, prosecutors were responsible for proving beyond reasonable doubt the defendant's sanity. Following reversion to the M'Naughten law, Congress placed the burden of proof of legal insanity squarely on the defendant, placed strict limitations on expert psychiatric testimony, and made hospital commitment and release procedures far more stringent. More than thirty states followed suit almost immediately. Some states completely abolished the insanity defense. As of 2002, Idaho, Montana, Utah, Kansas, and Nevada still did not allow the insanity defense, but Nevada later reinstated it.

Guilty but Mentally Ill

Subsequent to the more stringent requirements for an NGRI plea, many states adopted a new standard to make some kind of provision for the SPMI who commit a crime. The guilty but mentally ill (GBMI) plea was thus introduced. Under this verdict, the defendant is found guilty by a jury and sentenced in the same manner to the same form of punishment as any other defendant found guilty of that particular crime, rather than to commitment to a psychiatric institution. The only difference is that the finding of mentally ill entitles the defendant to treatment during incarceration. If the illness improves, the full sentence must still be served in a correctional facility. By 2000, at least twenty states had adopted GBMI laws.

Critics of the GBMI laws call it an oxymoron because it declares an individual guilty but not completely accountable, yet gives him or her the same sentence as if he or she *was* completely accountable. Critics also point out that the prison mental health system is generally completely unequipped to give SPMI people the type of treatment they need.

Who Should Decide?

Presumption of Competence: Because being accused of mental illness is similar to being accused of crime, we ought to presume that psychiatric "defendants" are mentally competent, just as we presume that criminal defendants are legally innocent. Individuals charged with criminal, civil, or interpersonal offenses ought never to be treated as incompetent solely on the basis of the opinion of mental health experts. Incompetence ought to be a judicial determination and the "accused" ought to have access to legal representation and a right to trial by jury.

Thomas Szasz, *Summary Statement and Manifesto, Point 3*
(Reprinted with permission from Dr. T. Szasz and www.szasz.com)

Many believe it is ludicrous to have jurors, who are uneducated in diagnosing mental illness, determine whether or not defendants claiming NGRI or GBMI are mentally competent. They point out that even psychiatrists cannot agree on the meaning of mental illness or to what degree an individual is mentally competent or incompetent. They also argue that the determination of competence occurs in an adversarial courtroom environment in which lawyers are pitched against psychiatrists—expert witnesses hired by the defense and prosecution—and psychiatrists are pitched against each other. Rather, a panel of court-appointed experts in psychiatry or psychology, who have no bias for either defense or prosecution, is far better equipped to evaluate an individual's mental competence and, as such, criminal responsibility. The facts of the case would then either proceed to the jury for a guilty or not guilty verdict as it pertains to the crime itself, or a plea could be made by the defense according to the panel's findings.

Others disagree with this perspective, arguing that psychiatrists are trained in medicine, not in law. Therefore, their expertise is in diagnosing and treating mental illnesses, which subsequently qualifies them to testify in court to the nature and severity of a defendant's condition when the crime was committed and to provide expert opinion as to why the defendant acted as he or she did. However, it must be the judge or jury, as society's representative, to legally determine criminal responsibility.

Szasz and others use an even more radical argument, believing that psychiatrists should not be involved in the legal process at all and that the verdict should be left entirely to the judicial system.

Regardless of arguments for or against jury determination of a defendant's mental competence, in an article in the March 17, 2000, *San Francisco Chronicle* by Katherine Seligman, Elizabeth Semel, who is professor of law at University of California-Berkeley's Boalt Hall School of Law and who runs the death penalty clinic there, notes that proving a defendant insane is virtually impossible: "There is huge chasm between our common-sense understanding of insanity and the legal definition of insanity. . . . The legal definition is an almost insurmountable standard."

Incarceration or Hospitalization

Of the SPMI convicted of a crime, most will end up in prison, even most of those who are found by a jury to be mentally incompetent. Is this the best option?

Proponents' Opinions of the Insanity Defense   Supporters of the insanity defense point out that following deinstitutionalization, the closure of most state psychiatric hospitals, and the general failure of CMHCs, the number of mentally ill in prisons has skyrocketed. The international human rights group Human Rights Watch found in 2003 that one in six prisoners in the United States suffered from some form of mental illness, particularly schizophrenia, bipolar disorder, and major depression, and that three times more mentally ill men, women, and children were in jail than in psychiatric treatment hospitals. The report also found prisons to be damaging and dangerous for mentally ill inmates, who are far more susceptible than other prisoners to mistreatment, neglect, and sexual and other types of abuse from both guards and inmates. Due to their illness, such prisoners find it virtually impossible to obey prison rules and are therefore often disruptive. Guards lack the necessary knowledge to differentiate between such behavior and prisoners who are deliberately disruptive. Therefore, the mentally ill are far more likely to receive harsher treatment, such as being placed in isolation, which often pushes them into acute psychosis. The report also found a serious lack of mental health services in many prisons, resulting in prisoners not receiving any form of treatment and a high rate of recidivism after release.

The number of SPMI prisoners on death row has also increased significantly, to an estimated 5–10 percent of the death-row population. In 1986, in *Ford v. Wainwright*, the U.S. Supreme Court ruled that under the Constitution's Eighth Amendment pertaining to cruel and unusual punishment, the insane cannot be executed unless they comprehend what the death sentence is and why they received it. Because many SPMI prisoners on death row do not meet these criteria, many states began providing them with treatment so that they *could* comprehend their situation and thus be put to death. International law prohibits executing a mentally ill person, and in 2000, the United Nations Commission on Human Rights urged all states that allowed the death penalty to not sentence to death any person suffering from a mental disorder. Although virtually every country in the world complied, the United States did not. According to Amnesty International's Web site:

- On January 6, 2004, the State of Arkansas executed Charles Singleton, who was said to be "seriously deranged without treatment" and "arguably incompetent with treatment." It was only during an episode of "drug-induced sanity" that the state scheduled his execution.
- On January 25, 2005, Troy Kunkle was executed in Texas although he suffered from schizophrenia and had a family history of mental illness.

Opponents' Opinions of the Insanity Defense   Those opposing the insanity defense argue that it is open to abuse by defense lawyers seeking an acquittal or a more lenient sentence who feel their clients have no better case. Some evidence supports this claim: after Connecticut doubled the amount of time that defendants acquitted on the insanity defense had to spend committed to a psychiatric institution, the number of insanity pleas decreased.

A longtime and outspoken critic of the insanity defense, Szasz believes that anyone who commits murder while in a psychotic state must be held fully responsible for his or her actions. Many agree with him. In light of his belief that mental illness is a myth, he declares that no one can be excused for breaking the law based on the opinion of a so-called mental health expert. Severely mentally ill criminals must be treated under the constitution as all other criminals, with the same constitutional right of trial by jury and the same punishment consequences.

Many argue that Szaz's philosophy is inhumane. Those who support him claim that incarceration in prison is more humane than incarceration in a psychiatric institution, where prisoners are subjected to forced treatment and traditionally serve longer sentences, with release always dependent upon the opinion of psychiatric experts and the facility's director.

PRIVACY VERSUS DISCLOSURE

What rights do patients have over their own medical information? Who owns the information—the patient or the provider? Do patients have the right to access and modify their information and to dictate who has access to it? Do providers have the right to share patient information with other providers without the patient's informed consent, particularly in the managed care environment? In the information age, how can patient confidentiality be ensured or enforced?

There is general agreement in the health care industry and the legal community that confidentiality laws are insufficient. The federal Health Insurance Portability and Accountability Act of 1996 (HIPAA) brought significant changes to legal and regulatory controls pertaining to security and confidentiality of individually identifiable patient health records in either written, electronic, or oral formats. Within the umbrella of federal laws, states have the right to implement their own laws, which vary widely. Reform measures, calling both for more rigid and for more lenient controls, are continuously being proposed at the national and state levels.

The confidentiality issue is particularly complicated where mental illness is concerned due to the extremely personal nature of the information that the client shares with the health care provider. Because of the stigma and discrimination that traditionally surround mental illness, loss of confidentiality concerning psychiatric treatment can be devastating for the client. Health care providers are permitted to disclose certain information to insurance companies in order to obtain payment; subsequently, employers who purchase health insurance for their staff may use the information contained in insurance records to terminate or otherwise discriminate against employees who have been treated for mental illness, and insurance companies frequently either disallow payments for treatment of mental health issues or terminate such an individual's entire policy. To avoid these situations, individuals will often either go untreated or pay for treatment out of their own pockets.

Disclosing information to a mentally ill patient's family is another controversial issue. In the case of adult children, some states allow caregiving parents or guardians limited access to information regarding diagnosis, treatment, and potential outcomes without the child's consent; some require the child's written consent; and others require administrative review if the child does not consent. Family advocates claim that a caregiving parent/guardian needs certain information in order to provide appropriate care. Concerns cited by health consumer advocates include the fact that conflicts within families could be exacerbated by disclosure and that the parent or family could force the child into treatment that is not wanted or needed.

According the 1999 surgeon general's report, *Mental Health: Report of the Surgeon General*, other controversial issues include the following:

- Oversight and public health reporting: All states allow entities with oversight responsibilities and public health officials to access health care records without a client's informed consent.
- Law enforcement agencies: Access by law enforcement officials to health records of people with mental illness is restricted in some states to situations when a crime has been committed at a treatment facility or when a hospitalized individual leaves without being discharged and does not return. Some states also allow law enforcement access to health records during investigation of health care fraud by the provider or institution.

  - Some reform proposals argue that broader access is particularly relevant to health care fraud investigations in which the provider, not the patient, is the issue. Others object on the grounds of privacy invasion and the possible use of treatment history in criminal cases.

- Disclosure to protect third parties: Following *Tarasoff v. Regents*, in which a 1976 California Supreme Court decision determined that a mental health professional is obliged to protect someone he or she believes is endangered by a client, all states now either mandate or allow such disclosure. Some states also release the clinician from liability if he or she does not take such action.

- Proponents agree on the grounds of constitutional police power or *parens patriae*. Critics object based on the constitutional issues of informed consent and individual rights, and note that such a decision to notify an endangered third party requires the professional to "assess future risk," something that is not always possible, and which is not legal in any other instance.

National Alliance on Mental Illness (NAMI): Advocacy Strategies and Goals Pertaining to Disclosure of Patient Information

1. Patient consent is the governing principle.
2. Consumers should be allowed to inspect and amend their health records.
3. Clinical information should be shared with families and caregivers.
4. States should be allowed to preempt the national standard with laws that are more protective of individual privacy rights.
5. The refusal by a consumer/patient to consent to sharing of clinical information shall not be used to deny treatment, adversely affect services, or otherwise discriminate against persons with severe mental illnesses. A patient's refusal to consent to the sharing of clinical information may however be a factor in determining whether or not medical negligence exists for clinical harms resulting from the non-exchange or the inadequate exchange of clinical information between providers.

CHAPTER 7

Treatment: When Does It Help? When Does It Hurt?

Amazing advances have been made in the treatment of mental illness, and scientific research into more effective treatments continues. Yet no treatment can prevent or cure mental illness, and no one seems to know why some treatments work for some people but not for others. Even how most treatments work remains somewhat of a mystery. Tens of millions of people have improved remarkably due to treatment; many have also died either from lack of treatment or because of it. One thing is certain: considerable controversy surrounds virtually every treatment modality for mental illnesses.

PSYCHOTHERAPY

As explained in Chapter 3, psychiatry is the science of the brain and psychology is the science of the mind—the latter focusing on mental processes and behavior. Within both sciences, but especially within the latter, treatment consists of psychotherapy in its myriad forms. Psychotherapy is a partnership between a client and a licensed and trained professional, such as a psychiatrist, psychologist, marriage counselor, social worker, or therapist. The objective of psychotherapy is to help clients to comprehend their feelings, worldviews, attitudes, and beliefs and to change those perspectives and behaviors as necessary to improve their life situation. With the development of brain-imaging technology, genetic research, and the ever-increasing popularity of psychotropic drugs came an increase in criticism of psychotherapy, and those practicing it strive to defend it as an effective treatment in any type of mental illness.

Criticisms of Psychotherapy

In his 1972 book *The Mind Game* (rev. Witchdoctors and Psychiatrists), research psychiatrist E. Fuller Torrey criticized techniques used by Western psychiatrists as being little or no better than techniques applied by witch doctors. In his 1978 book *The Myth of Psychotherapy: Mental Healing as Religion, Rhetoric, and Repression*, Thomas Szasz, himself a psychiatrist and perhaps the most outspoken opponent of Western psychiatry, accused psychotherapy of being a false religion that pretends to be a science that attempts to destroy true religion. He likened it to what once was called "curing of souls."

In her 1998 *SKEPTIC Magazine* article titled "Psychotherapy: Snake Oil of the 90s," Tana Dineen, a psychologist and author and a full member of the American Psychological Association and Canadian Psychological Association, opined that—as with witches' brew and the snake oil of traveling medicine shows—psychotherapy has no healing qualities and therefore is in many ways a scam. Dineen believes that just as the substantial amount of alcohol in snake oil made people feel better for a short time, so may talking to a licensed and, usually expensive, psychotherapist, but talking to a concerned, compassionate, and understanding friend is just as effective. She believes that long-term therapy is no more effective than short-term therapy, and in her 2001 book *Manufacturing Victims: What the Psychology Industry is Doing to People*, she accuses the psychology profession in general of creating victims through avenues such as marketing bogus psychological theories and therapies and fake cures while ignoring information that debunks their methods.

In 1999, freelance writer Ethan Watters and Pulitzer Prize winner Richard Ofshe, a professor of sociology at the University of California-Berkeley, published *Therapy's Delusions: The Myth of the Unconscious and the Exploitation of Today's Walking Worried* in an attempt to expose what they call the fraud of psychotherapy. This fraud, they believe, began with Sigmund Freud's assertion that although we may not consciously remember some things, our unconscious mind stores everything that ever happened to us, and we are therefore at the mercy of those unconscious memories. The authors disagree with this theory, the falsehoods of which they say has been perpetuated by the hundreds of different forms of therapy practiced in the present day. They criticize Freud's belief, also perpetuated by professionals in the field, that only trained analysts can understand how to reach and tame an individual's unconscious demons, thus ending problematic behavior through self-understanding and awareness. They also criticize the claims made by many psychotherapy professionals that even major mental illnesses can be cured in this manner. The authors accuse the field of psychotherapy of functioning with few checks and balances while building into therapy itself mechanisms to increase a client's devotion to it. In a 1999 interview with Salon.com, Watters said that after spending considerable time, money, and emotional energy with a therapist, it is extremely difficult for the client to abandon what he or she has come to believe is the "narrative that explains your life."

In his 2001 book *Common Sense Rebellion: Debunking Psychiatry, Confronting Psychiatry—An A to Z Guide to Rehumanizing Our Lives,* Bruce Lavine wrote, "From my experience with depression, it is always a psychological, social, and spiritual event, and providing morale for someone at a crossroads in his or her life is perhaps the most important thing one human being can do for another. . . . You can look for a talented morale builder among psychiatrists, psychologists, and social workers, but your chance of finding one will be better if you look almost anywhere else."

Among the many general criticisms of the profession are the following:

• Unless undertaken in a particular context, it does not adequately consider a client's culture, gender, race, or socioeconomic condition.
• Its individualistic nature supports dogmas that maintain the status quo of class and perpetuate gender and racial inequality and oppression.
• By talking about oneself and one's problems, it may encourage people to become self-centered.
• Time—particularly when accompanied by support from family, friends, peers, and clergy—as well as personal research and reading, contributes significantly to psychological and emotional healing.
• It is pseudoscience, a ritualistic enterprise that imitates the forms of science; psychiatric studies are based on subjective tests and opinions and psychotherapy is, at best, a questionable practice because it is unscientific.
• It is founded on philosophical worldviews, not on science. As such, what psychotherapy is differs between schools of psychotherapy and between individual psychotherapists within those different schools, as well as with changes in the worldviews themselves over time.

Defense of Psychotherapy

Proponents of psychotherapy argue that it is remarkably effective in decreasing depression, anxiety, and related physical symptoms, such as pain, fatigue, and nausea. The American Psychological Association (APA) suggests that the right match—between client and therapist—will do the most, by far, to ensure the best results.

In defense of the accusation that psychotherapy is unscientific, supporters argue that science means knowledge, and there are many fields of science, such as botany, mathematics, physics, and others, all of which are science in different ways. They declare that each science—including the sciences of psychiatry and psychology—should be defined by its own methods. Although critics suggest that the results of psychotherapy treatment cannot be tested scientifically, the APA declares that there is convincing empirical evidence that most people with emotional difficulties attending several psychotherapy sessions are far better off than individuals who do not seek treatment. Some proponents believe that in the broadest sense, psychotherapy is useful in all illnesses, even proving to be highly successful in many physical illnesses. They note that all physicians use at least a limited form of psychotherapy, even if just in reassuring a worried patient or encouraging treatment compliance. They point out that practitioners of psychotherapy are not only specifically trained in a variety of treatment modalities, they are also trained on when to use each modality. Their specialized training can help them understand a patient's specific needs, which allows them to define an individual structure for approaching each patient and to design treatment accordingly.

In general, therapy can guide an individual toward a solution to a difficult situation or problem by helping that individual gain a fresh perspective. Not everyone will be helped by therapy, just as not everyone is helped by medication. Therapy's success often depends on how willing and able the client is to become involved in the process and to apply the new information. Among the purported benefits of psychotherapy in its different forms are the following:

- Gaining greater self-knowledge, and discovering or understanding personal goals and values
- Developing relationship, stress management, anger management, communication, and problem-solving skills
- Overcoming specific problems, such as binge eating, alcohol or drug abuse, anorexia, anxiety, lack of self-confidence, etc.
- Resolving the issues that prompted one to seek therapeutic assistance

Psychotherapy in Depression
Of the many different modalities utilized in treating mental illness, the most thoroughly researched are those applied to one of the most prevalent disorders: depression. In general, the objectives of formal psychotherapy, particularly in the treatment of major depressive disorders, are similar to those of

medication: symptom relief, improved psychosocial functioning, and prevention of relapse and recurrence. Psychotherapy can take those goals even further by helping the client to address associated psychosocial problems, even if the symptoms of depression have been largely controlled with medication.

A fact sheet on the APA's Help Center Web site lists several ways in which skilled therapists can help individuals address or cope with depression by helping them to identify situational, behavioral, interpersonal, and psychological factors contributing to their depressed state. A well-trained professional can help the individual become aware of and define different options for emotional and cognitive responses to such factors, as well as assist the individual in developing specific psychological tools to develop positive responses.

Studies Supporting Benefits of Psychotherapy In a meta-analysis of several studies conducted by the Depression Guideline Panel of the Agency for Health Care Policy and Research (AHCPR), behavioral, brief dynamic, cognitive, and interpersonal psychotherapy alone were each found to be more effective than drugs alone in patients with depression (Figure 7.1).

A 1999 randomized, placebo-controlled trial conducted by Robin Jarrett at the University of Texas-Southwestern Medical Center at Dallas found that psychotherapy can be just as effective as monoamine oxidase inhibitors (MAOIs) in atypical major depression. In 2002, the University of Pennsylvania announced results of a 16-month study by Robert J. DeRubeis, professor and chair of psychology at the University of Pennsylvania, and Steven D. Hollon, professor of psychology at

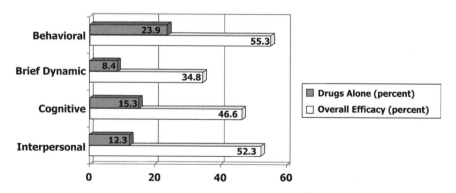

Figure 7.1
Meta-analyses of trials in outpatients with major depressive disorders showing efficacy of four types of psychotherapy alone compared with drug therapy alone. (Ricochet Productions.)

Vanderbilt University, that compared cognitive behavioral psychotherapy with medication in treating severely depressed people. The study focused on the best method to alleviate depression over the long term, rather than what would alleviate it most quickly. They found that—contrary to popular opinion in the psychiatric community—75 percent of patients participating in cognitive therapy did not relapse compared with 60 percent on medication and 19 percent receiving a placebo pill. They believe that even a short course of cognitive therapy may offer as much protection from depression as ongoing medication. In 2005, the same research team published results of another study in the *Archives of General Psychiatry*. They concluded that although it may depend on a high level of therapist expertise, cognitive therapy can be as effective as medications in the early phases of moderate to severe major depression.

Psychotherapy in Other Mental Illnesses

Psychotherapy has been shown to help in mental illnesses other than depression.

Drug Addiction   In 1989, G. E. Woody and coworkers published an article in the *American Journal of Psychiatry* after studying nonpsychotic opiate addicts attempting to get sober. The team found that psychotherapy added to drug counseling was more successful than drug counseling alone.

Anxiety Disorders   After studying the effects of psychoanalytically oriented psychotherapy with severely disturbed inpatients with anxiety disorders, in 1994, German doctors M. Bassler and S. O. Hoffmann published their findings in *Psychotherapie, Psychosomatik, medizinische Psychologie*. They found that

- 40.0 percent of patients with anxiety disorders improved; 21.2 percent failed to improve
- 61.4 percent of patients with agoraphobia improved; 6.3 percent failed to improve
- 52.5 percent of patients with panic disorder improved; 6.5 percent failed to improve

Schizophrenia   Because schizophrenia is now believed to have a biologically based component, rather than attempting long-term symptom relief, modern psychotherapeutic approaches to schizophrenia focus on short-term goals and skill acquisition. People with schizophrenia often make incorrect assessments of cause and effect, experience disorganized thinking, and often cannot learn from experience. Therapy addresses clients' ability to interpret reality and assists them in correct management of life problems. A 2000 review of several studies by Tracy D. Eells, published in the *Journal of Psychotherapy Practice and Research*, found that in general, the best results occurred with the combination of focused psychotherapy, medication management, and a stable living environment.

In the United Kingdom, where cognitive behavioral therapy (CBT) is used far more widely than in the United States, group CBT has been shown to considerably decrease positive symptoms (e.g., hearing voices) of schizophrenia. In 2005, Wykes et al. studied whether group CBT would also help alleviate hallucinations. Their results, published in *Schizophrenia Research*, indicated that CBT improved social functioning, but that reduction in hallucinations was directly related to receiving therapy early in the trial and to whether or not the therapy was provided by very experienced therapists who had been extensively trained in CBT.

Bipolar Disorder   In a 2003 article posted on the Medscape Today Web site, Deborah Spitz admitted that while there is a lack of systematic data regarding the efficacy of psychotherapy in bipolar disorder, there is support in the clinical literature that individual CBT and individual and family psychoeducational approaches help clients adhere to medication regimens, improve coping mechanisms when dealing with stressors, and improve social and occupational abilities.

Post-traumatic Stress Disorder   In 2005, a study led by A. K. Goenjian and published in the *American Journal of Psychiatry* found that grief- or trauma-focused psychotherapy after a natural disaster unequivocally has long-term benefits for adolescents. The team studied adolescents following the catastrophic 1988 Spitak earthquake in Armenia. They found that untreated adolescents exposed to the trauma were at risk for chronic post-traumatic stress disorder (PTSD) and depressive symptoms, and that even therapy that was provided 1.5 years after the earthquake and brief, specifically focused psychotherapy effectively reduced those risks.

DRUGS: A BRAVE NEW WORLD?

Tens of millions of people take drugs for these conditions, with differing degrees of success. When compared to placebos, the current
psychopharmaceuticals are certainly effective for some people, but
none are fully effective and all have side effects. Furthermore, psychiatric medications are misused and over-prescribed, while significant
underutilization poses its own problems. All these issues demonstrate
the need for better drugs.

Samuel H. Barondes, *Better Than Prozac*

In her report on the New York Academy of Sciences Web site, Mary
Crowley noted that Samuel H. Barondes, professor and director of the
Center for Neurobiology and Psychiatry at the University of California,
San Francisco, and author of *Better Than Prozac: Creating the Next
Generation of Psychiatric Drugs*, confesses that he is an "enthusiastic
fan" of psychotherapeutic medications, having prescribed them for
patients for more than 40 years, studied them in the laboratory, and sat on
advisory boards of biotechnology and pharmaceutical companies developing new drugs. He wrote, however, that while he has seen many excellent results with their use, he has sometimes seen miserable failures:
"Even the best of them are blunt instruments that have a large number of
effects on the brain, only some of which can be considered therapeutic."

Psychiatric Medication: Lifesaving or Life-Threatening?

Psychotherapeutic drugs have become the first-line treatment in most
mental illnesses, and the controversy surrounding their use remains contentious. There is also considerable criticism of what some believe to be
dishonest and unethical practices connected with drug approval processes
and with marketing by drug manufacturers.

Support of Psychiatric Medication As explained more fully in previous
chapters, psychiatric medications have proven effective for tens of millions of people and have often been hailed as miracles that allow people
with debilitating mental illnesses to lead happy, productive lives. Many
consider the increasing body of evidence to support hypotheses about the
biological underpinnings of many mental disorders. This evidence fuels
the hope and faith of researchers, clinicians, and clients alike that drugs
will become the answer to all mental illnesses for all people and may even
ultimately prevent them. New drugs are continually being researched,
manufactured, marketed, and prescribed in an effort to more safely and
effectively treat mental illnesses. At one end of the spectrum, some people

may find that without psychiatric medication life is difficult, yet they can still function relatively well. At the other end of the spectrum, others suffer psychological trauma, dysfunction, and disability to the point of needing hospitalization or of committing suicide if they do not receive the necessary medication.

Supporters of psychotherapeutic drugs argue that, even though drugs are not a panacea for everyone or for all mental illnesses, psychotherapeutic medication gives clients access to often life-changing and life-saving treatment, in many instances for disorders virtually impossible to treat with other therapeutic methods. This is particularly important in view of the fact that psychotherapy, often suggested as an alternative, is usually very expensive and coverage for it is often denied, or at best limited, by insurance programs.

Criticism of Psychiatric Drugs   Despite their benefits, the use of psychotropic drugs is heavily criticized. There is mounting concern about overprescription, particularly related to the use of antidepressants and drugs to treat attention deficit hyperactivity disorder (ADHD), and to their increasing use in children and adolescents. There is evidence—causing growing concern within the medical and psychiatric communities, in regulatory agencies, and even among the general public—that side effects that may be mild or virtually nonexistent in some people are serious or fatal in others. There are concerns regarding the seeming "quick fix" attitude of many doctors in prescribing psychiatric drugs and of patients in requesting them. There are concerns that antidepressants—which are very potent drugs—are increasingly prescribed by general practitioners untrained in the depth and nature of mental illness or in the effectiveness and dangers of such drugs, whereas mental health experts are specifically trained in both areas. There are concerns because the drugs address the symptoms but not the causes. There is the criticism that drugs simply suppress or provide an escape from unpleasant and painful, yet normal and important, human responses associated with anger, fear, grief, and other emotions, and that this suppression can be detrimental to both psychological and medical well-being.

Although certain mental illnesses respond to certain types of drugs believed to affect certain neurotransmitters (brain chemicals)—and there is mounting evidence to support the hypothesis of an underlying causal connection—as of 2006, there were still no concrete biological tests to evaluate neurotransmitter levels. Nor is it known with certainty how or why most drugs work. Those who oppose the use of psychiatric medication object vehemently to the fact that millions of men, women, and children are prescribed dangerous and potentially lethal drugs that have a multitude of effects on the brain, none of which are understood.

Antidepressants: SSRIs   The most widely prescribed antidepressants, and the most lucrative psychotropic drugs for manufacturers, are the newer drugs known collectively as selective serotonin reuptake inhibitors (SSRIs), with individual brand names including Paxil, Zoloft, and Prozac. Widely hailed by many, including many of those taking them, as being virtually miracle drugs, they are also widely blamed for severe and even fatal adverse reactions.

Is There a Link to Violence?   Violence, self-mutilation, and suicide are the most frequent reason for lawsuits against SSRI drug manufacturers. In particular, fluoxetine, the active ingredient in Prozac, manufactured by Eli Lilly, has been blamed for many violent acts and suicides. It is known that all SSRIs can act as powerful stimulants, which some believe causes *akathisia*, described in Lilly's patent of Prozac as being an inner restlessness. Some call it an inner torture, the likes of which probably never existed before the development of psychiatric drugs. It is believed that this neurological stimulation can be so powerful that it causes impulsive, violent behavior and suicide. Some theorize the stimulation can occur before depression is eased, thus giving the depressed person the energy or motivation he or she did not previously have to carry out such acts.

According to their "Report on the Escalating International Warnings on Psychiatric Drugs" posted on their Web site, the Citizens Commission on Human Rights (CCHR) claims that in 1990, they asked the Federal Drug Administration (FDA) and psychiatrists to issue warnings that the new-generation psychiatric drugs (SSRIs) could cause violence and suicide. In response, the FDA ordered formation of an advisory committee comprising nine psychiatrists, many of whom CCHR claims had financial ties with drug companies. Despite compelling testimony from medical experts, as well as individuals and families adversely affected by psychiatric drugs, nothing was done until 2004, when the FDA ordered drug companies to include a "black-box" warning on the packaging of the most popular SSRIs stating that they could cause suicidal tendencies in children and adolescents. Nine months later, the FDA issued warnings to physicians to watch for similar tendencies in adults taking the medications. According to CCHR's report, in the following year, approximately sixteen warnings were issued internationally about potential side effects, such as drug addiction and dependence, aggression, hostility, mania, psychosis, violence, and suicide.

In June 2006, a study by Michael Milane et al. published in the journal *PLoS Medicine* indicated that the use of antidepressants has saved thousands of lives. But the authors could not preclude the possibility of increased risk of suicide among small populations of individuals taking the drugs. The study analyzed U.S. federal government data on suicide rates from the early 1960s and Prozac sales from its introduction in 1988 through 2002. Although suicide rates remained relatively level for the 15 years prior to Prozac's introduction, they steadily decreased over the 14 years during which Prozac sales increased. Results suggested an overall decrease by 33,600 in expected number of suicide deaths since Prozac's introduction. While the authors acknowledged the yet unanswered question as to whether SSRIs increase suicide over and above the underlying major depression, they also acknowledged that many in the psychiatric community are concerned that lack of treatment may prove more harmful than the effects of the drugs. Julio Licinio, coauthor of the article, is quoted on the UCLA News Web site as saying: "Most people who commit suicide suffer from untreated depression. Our goal is to explore a possible SSRI–suicide link while ensuring that effective treatment and drug development for depression is not halted without cause."

Withdrawal Syndrome   Another contentious issue surrounding SSRIs are allegations of an often serious and debilitating withdrawal syndrome that affects some people going off the medication. This complaint has also resulted in litigation and class action suits. In regard to Paxil, Evelyn Pringle noted in an article on the lawyers and Settlement Web site that the World Health Organization (WHO) stated that it "has the highest incidence rate of withdrawal adverse experiences of any antidepressant drug in the world." Although the initial package insert mentioned the possibility of a withdrawal syndrome, those who pushed for stronger warnings claimed the existing one did not give a sufficiently clear picture to either doctors or patients as to the degree of difficulty or the length of time it may take to safely cease taking the medication. A new package insert recognized the more severe problems previously not acknowledged by the company, yet it did not admit that discontinuing the drug would cause such symptoms.

Other Side Effects   Manufacturers do warn about other side effects of SSRIs, of which sexual dysfunction is one common one. Yet critics still accuse drug companies of understating the rate of effects. In his controversial 2000 book *Prozac Backlash: Overcoming the Dangers of Prozac, Zoloft, Paxil, and Other Antidepressants with Safe, Effective Alternatives*, Harvard psychiatrist Joseph Glenmullen wrote that sexual dysfunction affects up to 60 percent of Prozac users, but Lilly admits to only 20–30 percent. In a 2002 analysis of liabilities faced by SSRI manufacturers published on the Harvard Law School Web site, Roger D. Rhoten wrote, "The inability of the drug companies to recognize and disclose the magnitude of side effects is magnified even more when looking at the fact that Eli Lilly's labels still indicated only a 2–5 percent occurrence of sexual dysfunction as of 2000."

Antidepressants: Bupropion   Bupropion, which is not an SSRI, is the active ingredient in the popular medications Zyban and Wellbutrin, prescribed primarily for depression but also often for weight loss or as a deterrent to alcohol consumption. It is the third leading cause of drug-related seizures, with cocaine intoxication being the first. Between 1998 and 2001, GlaxoSmithKline, Wellbutrin's manufacturer, received more than 1,100 reports of adverse reactions, including 172 seizures and nineteen deaths. In the United Kingdom, the Medicines Control Agency confirmed eighteen deaths and reports of adverse side effects from 3,457 patients in 2001 alone, yet the drug is prescribed even for children.

Antipsychotics

[T]oday we can be certain of only one thing: The day will come when people will look back at our current medicines for schizophrenia and the stories we tell to patients about their abnormal brain chemistry, and they will shake their heads in utter disbelief.

> Robert Whitaker, *Mad in America:*
> *Bad Science, Bad Medicine, and the*
> *Enduring Mistreatment of the Mentally Ill*

The general consensus among professionals in the psychiatric field is that psychotic, delusional, or manic states, particularly in schizophrenia and bipolar disorder, are virtually unmanageable without drugs. It is also generally agreed that schizophrenia should be treated with antipsychotics at the initial appearance of symptoms because delaying treatment may cause deterioration and brain damage. As a result, psychiatrists have been treating people earlier and more aggressively with antipsychotics, leaving, some argue, little opportunity to attempt other treatment modalities, such as closely supervised drug-free periods.

In 2005, John R. Bola published his results of a meta-analysis in *Schizophrenia Bulletin* in which he concluded that there is inadequate evidence that proves long-term harm from short-term postponement of medication. Bola's report quoted a Yale doctor who believes that although medication can be life-saving in a crisis, it may cause patients to be more deficit-ridden if continued and more susceptible to psychosis if ended. In a March 21, 2006, *New York Times* article about Bola's study, Benedict Carey noted that there have been several programs, including one in Finland and one in Sweden, that have successfully helped people cope with schizophrenia with minimal medication. He noted a significant factor, however: in contrast to the United States, the health care systems in both countries provide readily accessible psychotherapeutic services and inpatient care. Some experts, on the other hand, criticize Bola's report on the grounds that it is only one interpretation of the evidence and that not treating patients early and aggressively could prove dangerous to their future well-being.

Another issue with antipsychotics is their undesirable side effects. A large study conducted in 2005 found that over an 18-month period, three-fourths of people taking them became dissatisfied and discontinued treatment, and lawsuits claim that the use of Risperdal, Seroquel, and Zyprexa have caused health problems, including pancreatitis, diabetes, and stroke.

Psychotropic Drugs and Children   A major debate that began to develop in the latter part of the twentieth century concerns the escalating use of psychiatric medication in increasingly younger populations. In fact, a study by Thomas Delate et al. published in the April 2004 issue of *Psychiatric Services* indicated that the number of prescriptions written for psychiatric drugs for children is increasing by almost 10 percent a year (an almost 49 percent increase from 1998 to 2002), with the fastest-growing group of users being preschool children aged from 0 to 5 years.

Antidepressants   Between the late 1990s and 2001 in the United States, the number of antidepressant prescriptions for children younger than 18 years tripled, with more than 11 million prescriptions written for that age group in 2002 alone. Fluoxetine is the only antidepressant approved by the FDA for treating depression in children, yet others are prescribed off-label. As seen in the previous sections, considerable debate exists as to whether SSRIs in particular can trigger suicidal behavior in teens. Due to the debate—which essentially remains unresolved—and the black-box warnings, 2005 saw an almost 20 percent drop in antidepressant prescriptions for children. However, a major concern of physicians and many others is that children who remain untreated for depression are highly susceptible to suicidal tendencies and that the unresolved controversy may deter those who really need treatment from seeking it.

Antipsychotics   Likewise, the use of potent antipsychotic medications for children younger than 18, prescribed for difficulties such as aggressive behavior and severe mood swings, increased sixfold between 1992 and 2002. A study led by Mark Olfson, professor of clinical psychiatry at Columbia University College of Physicians & Surgeons, and published in the *Archives of General Psychiatry* in June 2006 found that in 2002, antipsychotics were prescribed to 1,438 out of 100,000 children and adolescents. Some scientists applaud the fact that children are getting the treatment they need, whereas others are concerned that children are being drugged simply for having normal childhood problems. Some attribute the massive increase partly to childhood difficulties now being given psychiatric labels previously reserved for adults, to increasing comfort levels among physicians with the new-generation drugs, and to more restricted access to psychotherapy and in-hospital care. Many child psychiatric experts believe that antipsychotics are the best method presently available to treat children in urgent situations who are nonresponsive to other modes of therapy. It should be noted that atypical antipsychotics such as Risperdal and Zyprexa have not been approved by the FDA for children; however, prescribing them is legal, and psychiatrists prescribe them for children off-label. Critics condemn the practice on the grounds that the drugs' mechanisms of action remain unknown, even in adults, and that the escalating use among American children is a huge experiment, often one of trial and error, in which their very lives serve as the research laboratory. Olfson commented on the use of the drugs: "They've been used in ways that haven't been as extensively studied and for which they haven't been approved by the FDA. . . . Whenever the practice gets out in front of the science, there's reason for concern."

ADHD Medication   ADHD, a behavioral disorder included in the *Diagnostic and Statistic Manual of Mental Disorders* (DSM) for the first time in 1980, is characterized by severe lack of ability to focus, inattentiveness, impulsivity, and hyperactivity. The disorder usually appears in early childhood, but it also affects adults. Much controversy surrounds the diagnosis and treatment of ADHD because no biological marker causing the disorder has yet been discovered, and diagnosis is entirely subjective. The disorder is primarily, and increasingly, treated with psychostimulant medications that stimulate the central nervous system. In what seems a like a counterintuitive response, the stimulants calm the overstimulation that appears to cause ADHD. Ritalin is probably the most well known of the many different ADHD drugs.

The National Center for Health Statistics found that between 1997 and 2002, the number of children in the United States aged between 3 and 17 who were diagnosed with ADHD increased by 1.1 million, and the number of children for whom ADHD drugs were prescribed increased significantly. The FDA announced in 2006 that 78 million such prescriptions were written between 1999 and 2003 for children ranging in age from 1 year (although no ADHD drug has been FDA-approved for children younger than 5 years) to 18 years, to the tune of $3.1 billion. Information from Medco Health Solutions, the nation's largest prescription benefit manager, revealed that from 2000 to 2003, the use of ADHD drugs in children younger than 5 years contributed to the overall increase of 23 percent for all children. Peter Breggin, author of *Talking Back to Ritalin*, believes parents, teachers, and doctors have been seriously misled by drug company marketing practices, to the detriment of America's children.

In a substantial article on OnlineJournal.com in April 2006, Evelyn Pringle noted that the debate over the deliberate drugging of children has been raging for years. "Schools have been accused of promoting the use of drugs to control normal but active children," she noted, and gave examples of testimony at a September 26, 2002, House Reform Committee hearing titled "Overmedication of Hyperactive Children." At the hearing, pediatrician Mary Ann Block testified: "Parents that come to me report consistently that the teachers and the principals and even the school nurses pressure them to go to a physician and get their child labeled and drugged. Some schools are giving lectures to parents, inviting parents to come hear talks about diagnosing and drugging their children for ADHD."

Many advocates of the use of such drugs claim that ADHD is a neurological disorder treatable with medication only and that the medication does not cause addiction or illegal drug use later in life. Others vehemently disagree. According to Pringle, Fred Baughman, neurologist, a leading expert in ADHD, and author of *The ADHD Fraud—How Psychiatry Makes "Patients" of Normal Children*, called current medical ideology surrounding ADHD a fraud: "one in which the FDA was fully complicit. . . . ADHD doesn't exist—it is not a physical abnormality, and as such bears no risk of causing physical injury or death as does every drug used in its treatment." When Baughman asked the FDA advisory committee panel of experts on March 22 and 23, 2006, to refer to any article that described any test that could be used to objectively prove that ADHD is a disease, no one could do so because, he says, there is no such test. Baughman told the panel that "informed consent demands not just a description of the drugs or surgery to be used but of the condition they are to be used on—

its prognosis and how that natural course/prognosis is likely to be altered by the treatments to be applied." According to Pringle, at the same hearings, it was noted that "no other countries are drugging children with stimulants." Also, psychiatrist Grace Jackson, author of *Rethinking Psychiatric Drugs: A Guide to Informed Consent*, testified that in 1996 and 1997, a WHO press release noted that 90 percent of all Ritalin's production and consumption occurred in the United States.

A February 2006 FDA report indicated that from 1999 to 2003, ADHD medications were attributed to twenty-five deaths, including nineteen children, and more than fifty instances of cardiovascular problems, including arrhythmia, palpitations, heart attack, stroke, and hypertension. The Drug Abuse Warning Network reported 1,478 emergency room visits recorded in 2001 related to Ritalin, an increase from 271 in 1990. The FDA also found there were almost 1,000 reports between January 2000 and June 30, 2005, of psychosis or mania possibly linked to ADHD medications, including Ritalin, Adderall, Concerta, and Strattera.

Concerns about the widespread use of ADHD drugs include the following:

- Adverse reactions such as agitation, irritability, anger, hostility, disinhibition, hypomania, mania, hallucinations, and psychosis
- Dangers involved if ADHD is inappropriately diagnosed
- Widely differing prescription patterns
- Off-label use in children under 6 years
- Excessive treatment duration

Summarizing some pertinent information in his book *Talking Back to Ritalin*, Breggin wrote on his Web site: "Our society has institutionalized drug abuse among our children. Worse yet, we abuse our children with drugs rather than making the effort to find better ways to meet their needs. In the long run, we are giving our children a very bad lesson—that drugs are the answer to emotional problems. We are encouraging a generation of youngsters to grow up relying on psychiatric drugs rather than on themselves and other human resources."

Psychotropic Drugs and the Elderly   There is a general perception among many—in the medical community and general population alike—that mental illness, particularly depression, is normal in the aging process. Many researchers and other experts, such as those in the geriatric psychiatry field, generally agree that this is not the case. They contend that because of the prevailing misconception, mental illness in the elderly is significantly underdiagnosed and undertreated. On the other hand, overuse and misuse of psychiatric medication in the elderly in nursing homes remains a serious concern.

According to a consensus statement by Dilip V. Jeste, et al. published in the September 1999 *Archives of General Psychiatry*, almost 20 percent of the present elderly population has psychopathological illnesses, and that rate is expected to increase by nearly 22 percent as the population ages. The authors predict a 275 percent increase in psychiatric illnesses among the elderly from 1970 to 2030, in contrast to a 67 percent increase among those aged 30 to 34. The authors also indicate that older people are susceptible to problems from prescription drugs for medical illnesses because aging affects the way in which people metabolize medication. Those problems often manifest as psychiatric illnesses.

Experts warn, however, about the dangers of using psychotropic medications for the elderly, particularly in light of the increased incidence of unwanted side effects over that in younger people. One particular issue is the safety of antipsychotics. The FDA mandated that the newer drugs, such as Abilify and Clozaril, carry a black-box warning stating that they almost double the risk of death in older adults compared with placebo. However, in December 2005, a study by a research group led by Philip Wang, published in the *New England Journal of Medicine*, found that older antipsychotic medications, such as Thorazine and Haldol, seem to be no safer and, in fact, may even be more dangerous, than the newer medications in the elderly.

Undertreatment or Overtreatment? Treatment for mental illnesses such as depression, anxiety, or paranoia has proven to be just as effective in the elderly as in the younger population. Yet dissension surrounding the topic persists. On the one hand, many professionals maintain that undertreatment in the elderly contributes significantly to inappropriate or premature admittance to nursing homes and to the high suicide rate among the elderly and elderly men in particular. The American Geriatrics Society (AGS) is among the advocates contending that mental illness in the elderly has traditionally been ignored and neglected and that even in light of the large numbers of individuals with Alzheimer's disease and dementia, research funding for mental illnesses in the elderly remains inadequate. It is of note that the Mental Health Parity Act of 1996 made access to mental health insurance benefits virtually impossible for millions of elderly Americans because of its limited scope and many exceptions.

On the other hand, there are accusations of psychiatric drugs being overused and misused among residents of geriatric nursing homes as a form of chemical restraint. On the Web site Mental Health Abuse: Exposing the Crimes of Mental Health Practitioners, Jan Eastgate, president of CCHR International, wrote: "To psychiatrists old age is a 'mental disorder,' a for-profit 'disease' for which they have no cure, but for which they will happily supply endless prescriptions of psychoactive drugs or damaging electroshock treatment."

ISSUES CONCERNING DRUG MANUFACTURERS

There are also concerns surrounding the drug manufacturers themselves: Do they fully acknowledge and disclose all side effects of their medications to regulatory agencies, physicians, and the general public? Do their enormous marketing campaigns unduly influence or pressure physicians and the American Psychiatric Association (APA) to endorse and prescribe their products?

Safety Issues: Is Pertinent Information Withheld?

Related to the issue of the potentially violent side effects of SSRIs are accusations that drug companies withheld information about these side effects from the FDA and other regulatory agencies. In particular, Lilly, the manufacturer of Prozac, has come under fire. By 2000, Prozac was the most widely prescribed antidepressant in the world, with more than 35 million people taking it. Also by that year, more than 200 law suits in the United States alone had been brought against Lilly, blaming the drug for suicide or violence.

The first real evidence that Lilly may have withheld important information from the FDA about the adverse effects of Prozac became public when Leah R. Garnett published an article in the *Boston Globe* exposing previously undisclosed, confidential information obtained from internal Lilly documents. One such document was a 1990 memo stamped confidential, written by a Lilly employee in Germany to executives at the U.S. headquarters. The memo indicated that the company's safety personnel were receiving instructions from the corporate group (Drug Epidemiology Unit) to "change the identification of events as they are reported by the physicians. . . . Our safety staff is requested to change the event term 'suicide attempt' [as reported by the physician] to 'overdose.' . . . it is requested that we change . . . 'suicidal ideation' to 'depression.'". . . . I do not think I could explain to the BGA [German regulatory authority], to a judge, to a reporter or even to my family why we would do this especially on the sensitive issue of suicide and suicide ideation." Other information published in the article showed that 3 years prior to approval by the FDA, the BGA refused to approve Prozac due to Lilly's studies showing that nonsuicidal patients taking the drug showed a fivefold increase in suicide attempts and actual suicide than did those prescribed older antidepressants, and a threefold higher rate than patients taking placebos.

In 2005, other internal Lilly documents were anonymously sent to the *British Medical Journal*, in which Jeanne Lenzer subsequently published an article exposing the information. A 1988 Lilly research document found that, among other adverse reactions, 38 percent of patients taking Prozac in clinical trials compared with 19 percent on placebo experienced "activation," which, in labeling, the FDA links to violent and suicidal behavior. Peter Breggin, who serves as a witness for plaintiffs in trials involving SSRIs and who published an extensive report in the 2003/2004 issue of *International Journal of Risk & Safety in Medicine*, believes the 38 percent reported by Lilly to be low, as other symptoms of activation, such as panic attacks, mania, and hypomania, were not included. According to Lenzer's article, after learning that Lilly had excluded, among other information, seventy-six of ninety-seven cases of reported suicidal tendencies, David Graham, then associate director in the FDA's Office of Drug Safety, wrote in a September 11, 1990, memo that "because of apparent large-scale underreporting, [Lilly's] analysis cannot be considered as proving that fluoxetine and violent behavior are unrelated."

Lilly is accused of having denied for years Prozac's allegedly dangerous side effects. According to another *Boston Globe* article by Mitchell Zuckoff on June 8, 2000, Gary Tollefson, a Lilly scientist, made the following statement under oath at the 1999 trial in which Prozac was blamed for William Forsyth, a wealthy 63-year-old man, stabbing his wife to death then killing himself. Tollefson said, "there is absolutely no medically sound evidence of an association between any antidepressant medicine, including Prozac, and the induction of suicidal ideation or violence." Yet shortly before that trial began, the company began working on a new form of Prozac. They acquired exclusive rights to a patent from the drug manufacturer Sepracor in December 1998 for more than $20 million, contracting to pay another $70 million based on how well the new drug performed in clinical trials. (The agreement was eventually canceled by Lilly, apparently due to heart irregularities discovered during the trials.) Prompted by the new patent agreement, the *Boston Globe* investigated, which resulted in Garnett's May 5, 2000, article. It was found that documents submitted to the U.S. Patent and Trademark Office contradicted the company's public defense of Prozac. The document stated that the new drug, R-fluoxetine, would decrease several of the original Prozac's adverse effects, including "akathisia, suicidal thoughts, and self-mutilation . . . one of its more significant side effects."

Other documents also came to light, such as a 1984 letter to Lilly from the British Committee on Safety of Medicines, which, according to Sarah Boseley writing for the *Guardian*, reads in part as follows: "During the treatment with the preparation [Prozac] 16 suicide attempts were made, two of these with success. As patients with a risk of suicide were excluded from the studies, it is probable that this high proportion can be attributed to an action of the preparation." Another document revealed that in 1986, Richard Kapit, chief medical officer in the FDA's Prozac approval process, found disturbing evidence, to which the FDA did not give adequate attention. According to Rhoten, Kapit warned in his 1986 Safety Review that Prozac could actually make some depressed patients worse and suggested that the drug be labeled to warn doctors of this possible effect. The FDA did not follow this suggestion; meanwhile, Prozac labels in Germany, France, and Great Britain all warned about its stimulatory effects and that they could lead to suicide.

Do Pharmaceutical Dollars Influence Physician Diagnosis?

Because of the huge profits associated with SSRIs, drug manufacturers have been accused of pushing their wares as treatments for a multitude of less serious problems in order to bring everyone, including children, into the circle of those who can be treated with them. As a result, many— including many doctors—believe the drugs are being overprescribed.

In a 1999 *Psychology Today* article, Loren R. Mosher accused drug companies of pouring "millions of dollars into the pockets of psychiatrists around the country, making them reluctant to recognize that drugs may not always be in the best interest of their patients. They are too busy enjoying drug company perks: consultant gigs, research grants, fine wine and fancy meals." Mosher suggested that, at that time, drug companies were spending approximately $10,000 per year per physician to "educate" them on the benefits of their drugs.

Mosher also accused the APA, which represents most psychiatrists in the United States and has upward of 40,000 members, of tolerating undue influence from drug manufacturer's profits. She indicated that the companies pay huge sums in rent to display their products at national APA conventions, that the APA derives an estimated 30 percent of its budget from drug company advertisements in its numerous publications, and that it accepts large, unrestricted educational grants from drug manufacturers. Mosher believes such a relationship is dangerous in that psychiatrists and researchers, with the "unspoken blessing" of the APA, may feel indebted to pharmaceutical manufacturers and thus develop a bias toward drug treatment over other treatment modalities. He goes so far as to say that, collectively, "these practices aggressively promote reliance on prescription drug use—so much so that many people think drugs should be forced on those who refuse to take them." Mosher also wrote that the APA "supports the National Alliance for the Mentally Ill [NAMI], which believes that mentally ill patients should be coerced to take medication. I am appalled by this level of social control. Mentally ill people should be given a choice to have their illness treated in alternative ways."

In the same article, Frederick K. Goodwin responded that Mosher was reopening a 25-year-old argument, long since settled by the benefits so many patients receive from psychiatric medications. Goodwin noted that, rather than creating alliances, drug companies actually compete for market share, and that "clinicians seem to be able to sift through competing claims and counterclaims." He also contended that the development of new drugs is essential to improve treatment options, and that that process requires a "close working relationship between industry, government and academia. The procedures and safeguards needed to ensure the integrity of this process require continued discussion. But it needs to be conducted seriously."

The article also printed NAMI's response to Mosher's accusation that it supports coercive treatment: "NAMI believes that all people should have the right to make their own decisions about medical treatment, but is aware that some individuals with brain disorders such as schizophrenia and bipolar disorder may at times, due to their illness, lack insight or good judgment about their need for medical treatment. Involuntary treatment of any kind should be used only as a last resort and only when it is believed to be in the best interest of the individual, following a court hearing in which due process has been provided."

ELECTROCONVULSIVE THERAPY

More than 60 years since its introduction, ECT—often called electric shock therapy—is still the most controversial treatment modality for mental illness. Many patients testify to its lifesaving effect when all else had failed; others testify it is a terrifying experience that left them with detrimental, often severe, cognitive disabilities. An estimated 100,000 people annually receive ECT, mostly in psychiatric units of general hospitals and in psychiatric hospitals. Treatment consists of inducing convulsions via electrodes placed on the scalp, through which electrical currents ranging from 170 to 500 volts are delivered (see Figure 7.2).

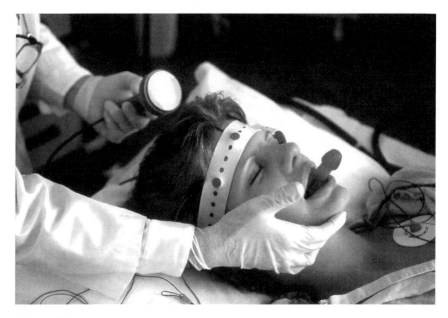

Figure 7.2
Sedated patient being prepared for electroconvulsive shock therapy (ECT). (Photograph by W. McIntyre.)

No one knows exactly how this makes depression lift. The treatment is endorsed by the psychiatric profession in general as well as by certain consumer groups. Proponents say it is the safest and best alternative in intractable cases. In his book *Bipolar Disorder: A Guide for Patients and Families*, Francis Mark Mondimore declared that ECT is perhaps the most effective treatment available for severe depression and severe mania, often taking effect more quickly than medication. Kay Redfield Jamison, author of *Night Falls Fast: Understanding Suicide*, recommends it as a first option over slower-acting medications and therapies to stabilize suicidal patients.

Opponents declare ECT is an inhumane and barbaric treatment modality often forced on unwilling consumers, and vehemently oppose its use at all, ever. They argue that it is ineffective, that it causes short-term, long-term, and permanent memory loss and brain damage, that it has high relapse rates, that it is increasingly used as a "quick fix" as opposed to hospitalization and/or long-term therapy, and that ECT experts are heavily biased. They also question why it is that the most enthusiastic supporters of ECT have never had the treatment, whereas the strongest opponents are those who have.

As seen in Chapter 3, the overuse and misuse of ECT in the mid-twentieth century brought it into serious disrepute, and its use declined substantially. In the latter part of the century, due to refinements in administration methods and the belief that it can be highly effective, it began to make a comeback. By 2006, it was even moving toward becoming the front-line treatment in severe bipolar disorder and depression.

Controlled studies suggest a 70–90 percent positive response rate to ECT; however, in clinical practice, the effectiveness of ECT and patient satisfaction with the outcome, or the lack thereof, varies among studies. In the June 2003 *British Medical Journal*, lead author Diana Rose published a review of twenty-six clinical studies conducted by clinicians and nine reports compiled by patients or with patient input. The review found persistent memory loss following ECT reported at rates of between 29 and 55 percent, with loss of autobiographical memory as the most commonly described, but inadequately investigated, side effect. The report concluded: "The current statement for patients from the Royal College of Psychiatrists that over 80 percent of patients are satisfied with electroconvulsive therapy and that memory loss is not clinically important is unfounded."

Another study, led by J. Prudic and published in *Biological Psychiatry* in February 2004, followed patients who received ECT in the clinical setting and also found a lower response rate than that indicated by clinical trials. Although methods varied between treatment sites, response rates were similar:

- 64 percent of patients responded to treatment
- 30 percent to 47 percent remitted
- 40 percent of treatment benefit disappeared within approximately 10 days
- 64 percent of 154 remitted patients relapsed within 6 months
- Predictors of poor outcome included comorbid personality disorder, longer duration of depression, schizoaffective disorders, and longer time before assessment.

According to the National Mental Health Association (NMHA), some researchers are adamant that benefits last no longer than 4 weeks. The NMHA also states that "During the last decade, the 'typical' ECT patient has changed from low-income males under 40, to middle-income women over 65. This coincides with changing demographics, the increase in the elderly population and Medicare, and the push by insurance companies to provide fast, 'medical' treatment rather than talk therapy. Unfortunately, concerns have been raised concerning inappropriate and even dangerous treatment of elderly patients with heart conditions, and the administration of ECT without proper patient consent."

A more damning accusation on the CCHR Web site reads as follows: "In the United States, 65-year-olds receive 360 percent more shock treatment than 64-year-olds because at age 65 government insurance coverage for shock typically takes effect. Such extensive abuse of the elderly is not the result of medical incompetence. . . . Studies show ECT shortens the lives of elderly people significantly. Specific figures are not kept as causes of death are usually listed as heart attacks or other conditions."

WHAT *IS* THE ANSWER?

Proponents and critics of different treatment modalities accuse members of the other side of bias, of exaggerating their arguments, and of choosing studies that reinforce their perspectives. Mental health consumers themselves differ in their opinions of each modality. Many people on both sides accuse drug manufacturers of putting profits before people. Regardless of perspectives and opinions, it appears that controversy surrounding treatment modalities will continue until scientific research finds definitive and indisputable causes for mental illnesses—if such causes exist—and develops safe, effective treatment—whatever form that may take—in light of such findings.

CHAPTER 8

Insurance: Who Pays and at What Price?

One of the greatest barriers to seeking treatment for mental illness is cost, and the availability of health insurance coverage, or the lack thereof, is one of the most important factors in determining access to mental health care. As seen in Chapter 1, untreated mental illness is enormously costly to the individual, the family, and the nation, yet the United States insurance industry has a long history of discriminating between mental and physical health benefits, always to the detriment of people with mental illnesses. As with physical illnesses, treatment for mental illness is expensive, particularly for the more serious disorders. Most employer-sponsored and state and federal plans provide only limited coverage for mental health treatment, and many *Diagnostic and Statistical Manual of Mental Disorders* (DSM-IV) diagnoses, such as substance abuse and dependence, are covered by very few plans.

Open discrimination—including denial of benefits for mental health–related expenses and even complete denial of all health care coverage—occurs against persons who acknowledge they have or have had a mental illness. Compounding the problem is the rapidly increasing poverty rate and number of uninsured individuals. In August 2005, the U.S. Census Bureau released its report on income, poverty, and health insurance, which showed that the number of people living in poverty rose by 1.1 million from 2003 to 2004 and that the number of uninsured individuals rose in the same period by 800,000, to 45.8 million. In the meantime, health care and health insurance costs continue to skyrocket, putting both out of the reach of millions.

PROTECTING PROFITABILITY AND INSURING AGAINST OVERUSE AND ABUSE

When designing insurance benefit plans, insurance companies try to protect themselves against *moral hazard* and *adverse selection*. The former is the concern that insured individuals who do not need to pay the full cost of treatment will use more services and that health care providers will recommend unnecessary procedures. *Cost sharing*, in the form of deductibles and copayments that must be borne by the consumer, and annual and lifetime limits on benefits reduce the moral hazard risk. To provide some protection for the patient, most plans set a *catastrophic limit*, above which the insurance company pays the entire cost of services. However, companies also protect themselves from unlimited expenses by setting annual and lifetime limits, above which patients or their family must bear full costs. Adverse selection is the concern that if one company provides more generous benefits that others, more consumers will choose that company, particularly those who need care the most, and thus benefit payouts will be much greater for that company. To protect against adverse selection, companies place restrictions on the types of coverage they provide.

INSURANCE DISPARITY

In 1999, the office of the U.S. surgeon general published its first-ever report on mental health, titled *Mental Health: Report of the Surgeon General*. This comprehensive report addresses past, present, and future issues surrounding mental health, including the disparity between physical and mental health insurance benefits. The report suggests that this disparity arose due to insurance company concerns about how to protect themselves against the high costs of treatment for serious and long-term mental illnesses. Due to such concerns, some private-sector agencies implemented far lower annual and lifetime limits, fewer in-hospital and outpatient therapy visits, shorter hospitalization periods, and higher copayments, deductibles, and other service fees in their coverage for mental illnesses. Others added further restrictions by limiting benefits to certain diagnoses only. Still others refused to offer benefits at all. An economic study published in 1998 by Zuvekas et al. in the *Journal of Mental Health Policy and Economics* revealed that a family in which treatment for mental illness costs $60,000 a year incurs approximately $27,000 in out-of-pocket expenses, whereas a family with equivalent medical and surgical expenses pays out-of-pocket expenses of approximately $1,500 and $1,800, respectively. A 1998 report by the Hay Group titled *Health Care Plan Design and Cost Trends—1988 through 1997* indicated that the number of health plans placing day limits on in-hospital care for the mentally ill increased from 38 percent to 57 percent between 1988 and 1997, and those restricting outpatient visits rose from 26 percent to 48 percent. In 2004, Medicare Part B provided that after paying a $100 deductible, a patient pays 20 percent of Medicare's approved amount for outpatient medical expenses, but the patient must pay 50 percent of the approved amount for outpatient mental illness expenses.

HEALTH INSURANCE SYSTEMS

The issue of health care coverage is highly complicated and controversial, and it becomes even more so in the case of mental illnesses. A confusing array of health insurance systems and plans exists, which can largely be grouped into three major categories: fee-for-service plans; managed care, including health maintenance organizations (HMOs) and preferred provider organizations (PPOs); and public-sector agencies, such as federal (Medicare/Medicaid) and state and local agencies.

Fee-for-Service Plans

Until the early 1990s, when managed care agencies began to predominate, the most widely used form of health insurance was fee-for-service plans, which were provided by companies such as Blue Cross/Blue Shield. Under these plans, the insured are almost entirely free to choose their doctor, hospital, and other providers, and are thus in control of their own health care decision-making. Insurance companies reimburse the independent health care providers for what is known as *usual and customary fees*, less the amount the insured is obliged to pay the provider, called a *copay*. This is done once a preset dollar amount is reached, which is called a *deductible*; until this happens, the patient usually must pay the full fee out of pocket. The amounts of the reimbursements for usual and customary fees are established by individual insurance companies according to what they believe a particular health service is worth, and if the provider charges more or will not accept the usual and customary fee, the insured must pay the balance. Copays and deductibles differ depending on the policy and are usually higher in fee-for-service plans than in a managed care program. Copays are typically 20% per service; deductibles may be anywhere from $100 per person per year to $10,000 or more per person per year in the case of "catastrophic coverage" policies. Policies with such high deductibles are primarily purchased by individuals not covered under an employer program and who perhaps cannot afford the high annual premiums charged for lower-deductible policies, yet wish to protect themselves against the high cost of a catastrophic medical necessity.

Managed Care

Managed care is a broad term encompassing many different types of insurance organizations. Managed care is used to control, or manage, the use of health care services, perhaps the most well known being HMOs and PPOs. It is a general term used to describe an entity that contracts with selected physicians, hospitals, and other health care providers and services; processes insurance claims; and performs the many other essential functions involved in health care delivery. All these services are then organized into one large group, the goal of which is to provide quality health care services, including preventive and educational services, while containing costs. Enrolled individuals must attend a provider (physician or hospital) within that organization.

An HMO can be succinctly described as an organization offering prepaid, comprehensive health coverage to their enrollees for a fixed period. HMO organizations contract with specific providers and pay them a fixed, or capitated, fee every month for every insured member in the plan, whether the member uses their services or not. The insured are required to receive authorization to see a specialist. Some HMOs develop physician networks, called Independent Practice Associations (IPAs), which must operate under the HMO's guidelines but do so on a fee-for-service basis. HMOs serve a huge range of consumers, such as corporate and group plans, Medicare and Medicaid, and the Federal Employees Health Benefits Program. They are the most restrictive type of managed care programs, limiting procedures, providers, and benefits. As of 2004, 414 different HMO companies existed throughout the United States, with more than 70 million enrollees. PPOs had more than 90 million enrollees.

The primary difference between HMOs and PPOs is that in a PPO, a network of providers offers services on a fee-for-service basis but at a reduced rate to members enrolled in the PPO. Members seeking treatment outside of that group of providers pay higher copays and deductibles and usually also pay the portion of the bill not covered by the plan's usual and customary limits.

Although managed care plans met with strong resistance from both the medical profession and the general public, by the 1990s, they overtook fee-for-service plans, increasing from 48% of all insurance enrollees in 1992 to 87% in 1999. In 2005, 175.7 million people were enrolled in managed care programs. Managed care led to major changes in mental health insurance with the creation of carve-out plans, a process by which the managed care insurer contracts with a separate insurance agency to provide specialized "behavioral" health care coverage. Although managed care began in the private sector, due to astronomical increases in health care

costs, Medicare and Medicaid, the largest providers of health care coverage in the United States, have also adopted managed care programs.
Nationwide enrollment in Medicaid's managed care program grew from
4.8 million in 1993 to 10.3 million in 1995, and from 1994 to 2005,
enrollment grew from 23 to 61 percent.

Managed care remains controversial. Supporters credit it with bringing
down costs of mental health care and therefore making it more accessible.
Soon after the big shift to managed care, the RAND Corporation, a
national nonprofit research and analysis institution, did a study of a major
West Coast employer who switched from fee-for-service to managed care
in 1991. The study found that even though the company's mental health
benefits increased under their carve-out program, costs decreased dramatically, by 41 percent, and continued a slow decline (Figure 8.1). The
major contributors to reduced costs were that fewer patients were hospitalized, and that those who were hospitalized were discharged sooner.

Critics accuse managed care mental health plans of putting profits
before people, in that many patients are denied the care they really need
due to the greatly reduced allowance of in-hospital treatment days and
outpatient treatment visits. Managed care mental health plans strictly control which health care providers the insured may use, and they determine

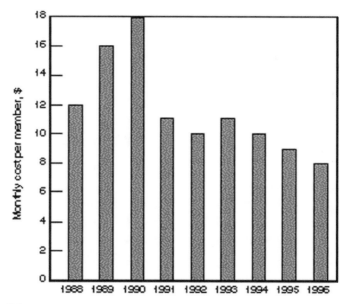

Figure 8.1
Mental health care costs decreased following the switch from fee-for-service plans to
managed care carve-out plans. (Ricochet Productions, after Rand Corporation, 1998.)

how much the provider is paid. Thus, neither patient nor provider is truly free to choose the type of care that may be optimal for the individual. Not only do these measures decrease a psychiatrist's or psychologist's autonomy in treatment planning, they encourage a move away from one-on-one talk therapy and intensive treatment. Instead, patients are referred to group therapy or prescribed medication for symptom relief, which in many cases may not address the root cause. Critics declare that treatment thus focuses on crisis intervention and stabilization and simply returns the patient to the state they were in prior to their emotional crisis, rather than focusing on addressing the root cause.

Managed care organizations, however, believe their plan design ensures accountability by both the patient and the provider, thereby reducing the risk of unnecessary or indiscriminate use of psychiatric services. As to restrictions on hospitalization, they contend that hospitalization should be reserved for patients who pose danger to themselves or to others and that hospitalization can make patients dependent, which tends to exacerbate the problems of people who are the sickest, as well as increasing their sense of institutionalization. In defense of limits placed on outpatient treatment and long-term, intensive psychotherapy, the insurance companies claim that denials are aimed not at those with severe mental illnesses, such as schizophrenia, but at restricting benefits paid for therapy that is undertaken for reasons such as interpersonal growth and the years of soul-searching undertaken by some patients and their therapists.

Medicaid

Federal agencies such as such as Medicare and Medicaid (the latter a complex structure that provides funds to states, under which each state administers its own program) provide a "safety net" for people unable to pay health care costs. Medicaid services the poor and underserved and, as such, is an important facilitator of mental health care, particularly as many seriously ill mental health patients are unable to work because of their disorders and are thus indigent. When Medicaid was enacted in 1965, replacing two other programs of federal grants to states, it adopted the Institutions for Mental Disease (IMD) exclusion, which specifically excludes insurance payments for patients in state psychiatric hospitals and other "institutions for mental diseases." Because a large portion of state and local government health care programs are funded by Medicaid, the IMD exclusion severely limits their ability to fund in-hospital psychiatric care.

Thousands of individuals were therefore released from state hospitals in an effort to get hospitalized patients off state and locally funded care and onto federally funded programs. In 1965, there were more than

500,000 patients in state psychiatric hospitals; by 1999, there were fewer than 60,000. Since 1955, more than 93 percent of state psychiatric hospitals have closed. There is no doubt that the development of psychiatric drugs, initially thought to be a "cure" for serious mental illnesses, contributed to this massive deinstitutionalization, but lack of funding was also a major factor. Although medication helped thousands of patients return relatively successfully to the community under the care of publicly funded community mental health centers (CMHCs), there were thousands of others who were released that medication could not help to do so. The result has been a huge homeless population, the extraordinary criminalization of the mentally ill, and increased victimization and violence toward them due to their vulnerability. Although conditions in many state hospitals may have been less than desirable, they did at least provide constant and comprehensive psychiatric, medical, and residential services for individuals who could not and cannot live independently and whose needs CMHCs are unable to meet.

Advocates of parity in mental health insurance may well support the policy analyst Bruce Rheinstein, J.D., who wrote in a 2000 *Catalyst* article titled "True Parity Means Eliminating Medicaid's IMD Exclusion" and published on the Treatment Advocacy Center Web site: "The primary question that drives the system today is not 'what does the patient need?' but rather 'what will federal programs pay for?'"

THE HIGH COST OF UNTREATED MENTAL ILLNESS

While insurance providers argue that they cannot afford parity for mental health benefits, advocates argue that the nation cannot afford to allow mentally ill patients to go untreated. Apart from the fact that billions of dollars of income are lost each year due to the inability of untreated, seriously mentally ill people to work, the social implications are enormous.

Homelessness

A 2005 study by the University of California–San Diego found that the rate of homelessness in persons with serious mental illnesses is 15 percent. Of the estimated 600,000 U.S. homeless, 200,000—one-third—are individuals with untreated mental illnesses. For these individuals, quality of life is appalling, and one study found that 28 percent of the homeless mentally ill obtain some food from garbage cans and that for 8 percent of the homeless previously in a psychiatric hospital, garbage cans are their primary food source.

Incarceration

An April 2005 article titled "Senators Press for Funding Mental Illness Criminal Justice Programs," posted on the National Alliance for the Mentally Ill (NAMI) Web site, reported estimates by the U.S. Department of Justice that upward of 300,000, or more than 16%, of all incarcerated people suffer from serious mental illnesses, many with coexisting substance abuse/dependency disorders. Rates in the juvenile justice system are even higher: recent studies indicate that one out of every five juveniles incarcerated suffers from a serious mental disorder. Many crimes committed by the mentally ill are misdemeanors, but many others are felonies most often caused by psychotic thinking. Mentally ill inmates who remain untreated are incarcerated twice as long and are twice as likely to commit suicide as are healthy inmates.

Violent Acts

Of the approximately 20,000 homicides in the United States annually, an estimated 1,000 are perpetrated by people with untreated schizophrenia or manic-depressive disorder. According to a fact sheet titled "Consequences of Non-Treatment" and posted on the Treatment Advocacy Center Web site, a 1998 study by the MacArthur Foundation reported that individuals with serious brain disorders committed twice as many violent acts immediately prior to their hospitalization and treatment than they did after hospitalization and while continuing to receive the necessary treatment.

Suicide

Close to 30,000 suicide deaths occur each year in the United States, of which at least 5,000 are individuals who had schizophrenia or bipolar disorder, most of whom were not receiving adequate psychiatric treatment at the time of death.

PUSHING FOR PARITY

For the above reasons and many more, advocates from both the private and the public sectors have long been pushing for insurance parity between physical and mental illness. As a result, some legislation has been implemented on both federal and state levels in the form of parity acts. Nevertheless, advocate groups and those with mental disorders believe legislation falls far short of the desired goals.

Mental Health Parity Act of 1996

On September 26, 1996, President Bill Clinton signed into law the federal government's Mental Health Parity Act of 1996 (MHPA), a landmark law that received overwhelming political support. The intent of this act was to end insurance companies' discriminatory practices of providing fewer benefits for mental illnesses than for equally serious physical illnesses. The act took effect in January 1998 and expired on September 30, 2001. However, it was extended five times and, as of 2006, was scheduled to expire on December 31 that year. Following is a 1996 summary of the act, provided on the NAMI Web site:

- The law equates aggregate [cumulative] lifetime limits and annual limits for mental health benefits with aggregate lifetime limits and annual limits for medical and surgical benefits. *(Typical caps for mental illness coverage are $50,000 for lifetime and $5,000 for annual, as compared with $1 million lifetime and no annual cap for other physical disorders.)*
- The law covers mental illnesses (i.e., "mental health services," as defined under the terms of individual plans); it does not cover treatment of substance abuse or chemical dependency.
- Existing state parity laws are not preempted by the federal law *(i.e., a state law requiring more comprehensive coverage would not be weakened by the federal law, nor does it preclude a state from enacting stronger parity legislation).*
- The law applies only to employers that offer mental health benefits; it does not mandate such coverage.
- The law allows for many cost-shifting mechanisms, such as adjusting limits on mental illness inpatient days, prescription drugs, outpatient visits, raising co-insurance and deductibles, and modifying the definition of medical necessity. *(Therefore, lower limits for inpatient and outpatient mental illness treatments are expected to continue, and in some cases, actually expand to help keep costs down.)*
- The law applies both to fully insured state-regulated health plans and to self-insured plans that are exempt from state laws under the Employee Retirement Income Security Act (ERISA), which are regulated by the Department of Labor.
- The law has a small business exemption, which excludes businesses with fifty employees or less.
- The law allows an increased cost exemption; employers that can demonstrate a one percent or more rise in costs due to parity implementation will be allowed to exempt themselves from the law.

The act did not designate a minimum number of inpatient days or outpatient consultations that must be covered, nor did it restrict the authority of an insurance plan to manage the care a patient receives, nor does it apply to Medicare or Medicaid. Loopholes allow companies to circumvent the law, and thus true parity is not ensured. However, some feel that the act does benefit individuals with the most severe, long-term, and disabling brain disorders, because they are more likely to exceed the lower annual and lifetime limits once imposed for mental health care coverage.

The act brought about some improvements, including—according to Bureau of Labor Statistics report published in 2003—that among companies employing 100 or more individuals, there was a significant decrease in the number imposing dollar limits on care received: the number of workers with dollar limits on inpatient care dropped from 41 percent in 1997 to 10 percent in 2000, and those with outpatient care limits dropped from 55 percent to 15 percent. Prior to the act, only five states had parity legislation, but that number increased to twenty-eight after the act. Some states even imposed more stringent regulations against discrimination than did the federal act.

Arguments against Parity

Opponents of parity legislation, primarily insurance companies, point out that because mental illnesses are not diagnosable by physical tests and therefore are based solely observation, diagnoses are arbitrary and depend upon the diagnosing physician. Therefore, mental health providers can define new illnesses without any scientific basis. These scenarios could lead to insurance abuse through insurance claims that are not confirmable.

Another argument is that mentally ill patients are often treated or hospitalized against their will by health care professionals who then file claims for the unwanted and expensive treatments. This was a particular scandal in the 1980s and early 1990s. They also argue that millions of people are prescribed dozens of new and expensive psychiatric drugs, yet scientific evidence does not indicate that either the incidence or the prevalence of mental illnesses has decreased, or even that long-term outcomes have improved over older medications.

Further concerns include the following:

- Employer costs and worker premiums for insurance coverage will increase significantly
- Parity without managed care is like giving providers a blank check
- Legislation enforcing coverage for all DSM-IV diagnoses and treatment would lead to coverage of hundreds of questionable disorders
- Government mandates for parity are just another attempt toward expanding regulation of health care benefits and business pay practices.

Arguments in Favor of Parity

In an article on their Web site titled "Why Mental Health Parity Makes Economic Sense," the National Mental Health Association (NMHA) Healthcare Reform Advocacy Resource Center presented the following arguments for parity gleaned from a number of studies:

Without Parity, We Waste Money

- The combined indirect and related costs of mental illness, including costs of lost productivity, lost earnings due to illness, and social costs. are estimated to total at least $113 billion annually.
- Clinical depression alone costs the United States $43.7 billion annually, including workplace costs for absenteeism and lost productivity ($23.8 billion), direct cots for treatment and rehabilitation ($12.4 billion), and lost earning due to depression-induced suicides ($7.5 billion).
- Health plans with the highest financial barriers to mental health services have higher rates of psychiatric long-term disability (LTD) claims, and companies with easier access to mental health services see a reduced incidence of LTD claims.
- Cutting dollars for mental health care can increase overall medical costs. A 30 percent cost reduction in mental health services at a large Connecticut corporation triggered a 37 percent increase in medical care use and sick leave by employees using mental health services, thus costing the corporation more money, rather than saving it money.
- Health care costs of untreated persons who suffer from alcohol and drug addiction are 100 percent higher than those of persons who receive treatment. Of all hospital admissions, at least 25 percent of those admitted suffer from alcoholism-related complications, and 65 percent of emergency room visits are alcohol- or otherwise drug-related.

Parity Is Affordable

- Introducing mental health parity in conjunction with managed care results in a 30 to 50 percent decrease in total mental health costs. In systems that are already using managed care, implementing parity results in a less than one percent increase in health care costs.
- It is estimated that parity would increase premiums by only 1.4 to 1.6 percent, and warned that this estimate may still be too high.

- "Employers have not attempted to avoid parity laws by becoming self-insured, and they do not tend to pass on the costs of parity to employees. The low cost of adopting parity allows employers to keep employee health care contributions at the same level they were before parity."
- SAMHSA [Substance Abuse and Mental Health Services Association] estimates that severe mental illnesses (biologically based illnesses) account for 90 percent of any cost increases from parity. They further estimate that adding children to federal legislation would result in a cost increase of approximately 0.8 percent in managed care settings.
- In Minnesota, Blue Cross/Blue Shield reduced its insurance premiums by five to six percent after one year's experience under the state's comprehensive parity law.
- In North Carolina, mental health expenses have decreased every year since comprehensive parity for state and local employees was passed in 1992. Mental health costs, as a percentage of total health benefits, have decreased from 6.4 percent in 1992 to 3.1 percent in 1998. Since 1992, hospital days paid by the plan have been reduced by 70 percent.

Parity Improves Access to Services and Saves Money

- While the estimated annual cost to the nation of providing mental health coverage commensurate to physical health coverage for all children and adults is $6.5 billion, it is also estimated that this mental health coverage would result in savings for general medical services and indirect costs in the amount of $8.7 billion—*a net annual savings of $2.2 billion.*
- Studies have found that overall medical care costs decrease for those using behavioral health care services, when such costs were generally increasing.
- Employment Assistance Programs (EAPs) have proven to be cost-effective. Chevron saved seven dollars for every dollar it spent on its EAP; Campbell Soup Company had a 28 percent reduction in mental health care costs; and Virginia Power realized a 23 percent drop in medical claims over a four-year period for individuals who accessed the EAP, compared with those who accessed behavioral health benefits on their own.
- At McDonnell Douglas, absenteeism dropped 44 percent for employees treated for substance abuse issues, and they set the

three-year value of employee assistance services at $4.4 million in medical claims. When the Kennecott Copper Corporation provided mental health counseling for employees, its hospital, medical, and surgical costs decreased 48.9 percent.

Some other arguments for the need for insurance parity are as follows:

- State and local government financing provides something of a "safety net" for the indigent mentally ill.
- Huge gaps in continuity of treatment exist between the different systems, and administrative costs are duplicated.
- Coverage limited to "severe mental illnesses" is like limiting physical care to severe illnesses; it discriminates against children, adolescents, and all whose illness does not meet the "severe criteria" defined by insurance companies; and many disorders often excluded—such as anorexia, bulimia, post-traumatic stress syndrome, multiple personality disorders, and substance abuse—can be just as debilitating as those defined by insurance companies as severe. For example, in 2005, alcohol and drug addictions—designated as a mental illness in the DSM-IV-TR—that remain untreated cost taxpayers $400 billion.
- Life insurance and income protection are difficult for the mentally ill to obtain, payments are often denied, and policies are sometimes even canceled when claims are made.

The surgeon general's report states the following:

Concerns about the cost of care—concerns made worse by the disparity in insurance coverage for mental disorders in contrast to other illnesses—are among the foremost reasons why people do not seek needed mental health care. While both access to and use of mental health services increase when benefits for those services are enhanced, preliminary data show that the effectiveness—and, thus, the value—of mental health care also has increased in recent years, while expenditures for services, under managed care, have fallen. Equality between mental health coverage and other health coverage—a concept known as parity—is an affordable and effective objective.

SECTION THREE

References and Resources

Annotated Primary Documents

APPENDIX ITEM I: EXCERPTS FROM THE SECOND U.S. SURGEON GENERAL'S REPORT ON MENTAL HEALTH AND MENTAL ILLNESS

This report addresses discrimination issues experienced by mentally ill members of certain minority groups. It is notable, however, that between 1964 and 2004, the surgeon general released twenty-eight reports on smoking as it relates to health. Despite the well-recognized, devastating effects of mental illness on individuals and families and its huge burden on society, mental illness was first addressed by the surgeon general in 1999 in the report *Mental Health: A Report of the Surgeon General*, which has been referred to in the text. In 2001, the surgeon general released a supplement to that report addressing the serious discrimination experienced by certain minorities with mental illnesses. As noted in the report's "Executive Summary," many other minorities with mental illnesses—such as people who are gay, lesbian, bisexual, and transgendered, or those with comorbid physical illnesses—are not specifically addressed; however, most conclusions drawn by the study apply just as readily to those individuals. To access the references cited in the report, please go to the References link at http://www.surgeongeneral.gov/library/mentalhealth/cre/execsummary-7.html.

Culture, Race, and Ethnicity. A Supplement to Mental Health: A Report of the Surgeon General

Main Findings

Mental Illnesses are Real, Disabling Conditions Affecting All Populations, Regardless of Race or Ethnicity Major mental disorders like schizophrenia, bipolar disorder, depression, and panic disorder are found worldwide, across all racial and ethnic groups. They have been found across the globe, wherever researchers have surveyed. In the United States, the overall annual prevalence of mental disorders is about 21 percent of adults and children (DHHS, 1999). This Supplement finds that, based on the available evidence, the prevalence of mental disorders for racial and ethnic minorities in the United States is similar to that for whites.

This general finding about similarities in overall prevalence applies to minorities living in the community. It does not apply to those individuals in vulnerable, high-need subgroups such as persons who are homeless, incarcerated, or institutionalized. People in these groups have higher rates of mental disorders (Koegel et al., 1988; Vernez et al., 1988; Breakey et al., 1989; Teplin, 1990). Further, the rates of mental disorders are not sufficiently studied in many smaller racial and ethnic groups—most notably American Indians, Alaska Natives, Asian Americans, and Pacific Islander groups—to permit firm conclusions about overall prevalence within those populations.

This Supplement pays special attention to vulnerable, high-need populations in which minorities are overrepresented. Although individuals in these groups are known to have a high need for mental health care, they often do not receive adequate services. This represents a critical public health concern, and this Supplement identifies as a course of action the need for earlier identification and care for these individuals within a coordinated and comprehensive service delivery system.

Most epidemiological studies using disorder-based definitions of mental illness are conducted in community household surveys. They fail to include nonhousehold members, such as persons without homes, or persons residing in institutions such as residential treatment centers, jails, shelters, and hospitals.

Striking Disparities in Mental Health Care Are Found for Racial and Ethnic Minorities This Supplement documents the existence of several disparities affecting mental health care of racial and ethnic minorities compared with whites:

- Minorities have less access to, and availability of, mental health services.
- Minorities are less likely to receive needed mental health services.
- Minorities in treatment often receive a poorer quality of mental health care.
- Minorities are underrepresented in mental health research.

The recognition of these disparities brings hope that they can be seriously addressed and remedied. This Supplement offers guidance on future courses of action to eliminate these disparities and to ensure equality in access, utilization, and outcomes of mental health care.

More is known about the disparities than the reasons behind them. A constellation of barriers deters minorities from reaching treatment. Many of these barriers operate for all Americans: cost, fragmentation of services, lack of availability of services, and societal stigma toward mental illness (DHHS, 1999). But additional barriers deter racial and ethnic minorities; mistrust and fear of treatment, racism and discrimination, and differences in language and communication. The ability for consumers and providers to communicate with one another is essential for all aspects of health care, yet it carries special significance in the area of mental health because mental disorders affect thoughts, moods, and the highest integrative aspects of behavior. The diagnosis and treatment of mental disorders greatly depend on verbal communication and trust between patient and clinician. More broadly, mental health care disparities may also stem from minorities' historical and present day struggles with racism and discrimination, which affect their mental health and contribute to their lower economic, social, and political status. The cumulative weight and interplay of all barriers to care, not any single one alone, is likely responsible for mental health disparities.

Although a number of terms identify people who use or have used mental health services (e.g., mental health consumer, survivor, ex-patient, client), the terms "consumer" and "patient" will be used interchangably throughout this Supplement.

Disparities Impose a Greater Disability Burden on Minorities   This Supplement finds that racial and ethnic minorities collectively experience a greater disability burden from mental illness than do whites. This higher level of burden stems from minorities receiving less care and poorer quality of care, rather than from their illnesses being inherently more severe or prevalent in the community.

This finding draws on several lines of evidence. First, mental disorders are highly disabling for all the world's populations (Murray & Lopez, 1996; Druss et al., 2000). Second, minorities are less likely than whites to receive needed services and more likely to receive poor quality of care. By not receiving effective treatment, they have greater levels of disability in terms of lost workdays and limitations in daily activities. Further, minorities are overrepresented among the Nation's most vulnerable populations, which have higher rates of mental disorders and more barriers to care. Taken together, these disparate lines of evidence support the finding that minorities suffer a disproportionately high disability burden from unmet mental health needs.

The greater disability burden is of grave concern to public health, and it has very real consequences. Ethnic and racial minorities do not yet completely share in the hope afforded by remarkable scientific advances in understanding and treating mental disorders. Because of disparities in mental health services, a disproportionate number of minorities with mental illnesses do not fully benefit from, or contribute to, the opportunities and prosperity of our society. This preventable disability from mental illness exacts a high societal toll and affects all Americans. Most troubling of all, the burden for minorities is growing. They are becoming more populous, all the while experiencing continuing inequality of income and economic opportunity. Racial and ethnic minorities in the United States face a social and economic environment of inequality that includes greater exposure to racism and discrimination, violence, and poverty, all of which take a toll on mental health.

[Following is the report's summary of Chapter 2]:

Chapter Summaries & Conclusions

Chapter 2: Culture Counts   The cultures of racial and ethnic minorities influence many aspects of mental illness, including how patients from a given culture communicate and manifest their symptoms, their style of coping, their family and community supports, and their willingness to seek treatment. Likewise, the cultures of the clinician and the service system influence diagnosis, treatment, and service delivery. Cultural and social influences are not the only determinants of mental illness and patterns of service use, but they do play important roles.

- Cultural and social factors contribute to the causation of mental illness, yet that contribution varies by disorder. Mental illness is considered the product of a complex interaction among biological, psychological, social, and cultural factors. The role of any of these major factors can be stronger or weaker depending on the specific disorder.

- Ethnic and racial minorities in the United States face a social and economic environment of inequality that includes greater exposure to racism, discrimination, violence, and poverty. Living in poverty has the most measurable effect on the rates of mental illness. People in the lowest strata of income, education, and occupation (known as socioeconomic status) are about two to three times more likely than those in the highest strata to have a mental disorder.

- Racism and discrimination are stressful events that adversely affect health and mental health. They place minorities at risk for mental disorders such as depression and anxiety. Whether racism and discrimination can by themselves cause these disorders is less clear, yet deserves research attention.

- Mistrust of mental health services is an important reason deterring minorities from seeking treatment. Their concerns are reinforced by evidence, both direct and indirect, of clinician bias and stereotyping.

- The cultures of racial and ethnic minorities alter the types of mental health services they need. Clinical environments that do not respect, or are incompatible with, the cultures of the people they serve may deter minorities from using services and receiving appropriate care.

APPENDIX ITEM II: DR. THOMAS SZASZ'S *SUMMARY STATEMENT AND MANIFESTO*

Szasz (1920–), Professor Emeritus in Psychiatry at the State University of New York's Health Science Center, is perhaps most famous for his controversial books *The Myth of Mental Illness* and *The Manufacture of Madness: A Comparative Study of the Inquisition and the Mental Health Movement*. Although incorrectly often associated with the antipsychiatry movement, he does not argue against psychiatry but against the way it is too frequently misused. The major premise of his viewpoint is that each individual has the right to self-ownership, be it physical or mental, and the right to be free of violence from others. Szasz and others who adhere to his philosophies believe that, whether or not one believes in the existence of mental illness, psychiatry must only be practiced between consenting adults, with no state interference or coercion. This manifesto, reprinted here with permission from Dr. T. Szasz and www.szasz.com, can be accessed at http://www.szasz.com/manifesto.html.

Thomas Szasz's Summary Statement and Manifesto

1. *"Myth of mental illness."* Mental illness is a metaphor (metaphorical disease). The word "disease" denotes a demonstrable biological process that affects the bodies of living organisms (plants, animals, and humans). The term "mental illness" refers to the undesirable thoughts, feelings, and behaviors of persons. Classifying thoughts, feelings, and behaviors as diseases is a logical and semantic error, like classifying the whale as a fish. As the whale is not a fish, mental illness is not a disease. Individuals with brain diseases (bad brains) or kidney diseases (bad kidneys) are literally sick. Individuals with mental diseases (bad behaviors), like societies with economic diseases (bad fiscal policies), are metaphorically sick. The classification of (mis)behavior as illness provides an ideological justification for state-sponsored social control as medical treatment.

2. *Separation of Psychiatry and the State.* If we recognize that "mental illness" is a metaphor for disapproved thoughts, feelings, and behaviors, we are compelled to recognize as well that the primary function of Psychiatry is to control thought, mood, and behavior. Hence, like Church and State, Psychiatry and the State ought to be separated by a "wall." At the same time, the State ought not to interfere with mental health practices between consenting adults. The role of psychiatrists and mental health experts with regard to law, the school system, and other organizations ought to be similar to the role of clergymen in those situations.

3. *Presumption of competence.* Because being accused of mental illness is similar to being accused of crime, we ought to presume that psychiatric "defendants" are mentally competent, just as we presume that criminal defendants are legally innocent. Individuals charged with criminal, civil, or interpersonal offenses ought never to be treated as incompetent solely on the basis of the opinion of mental health experts. Incompetence ought to be a judicial determination and the "accused" ought to have access to legal representation and a right to trial by jury.

4. *Abolition of involuntary mental hospitalization.* Involuntary mental hospitalization is imprisonment under the guise of treatment; it is a covert form of social control that subverts the rule of law. No one ought to be deprived of liberty except for a criminal offense, after a

trial by jury guided by legal rules of evidence. No one ought to be detained against his will in a building called "hospital," or in any other medical institution, or on the basis of expert opinion. Medicine ought to be clearly distinguished and separated from penology, treatment from punishment, the hospital from the prison. No person ought to be detained involuntarily for a purpose other than punishment or in an institution other than one formally defined as a part of the state's criminal justice system.

5. *Abolition of the insanity defense.* Insanity is a legal concept involving the courtroom determination that a person is not capable of forming conscious intent and, therefore, cannot be held responsible for an otherwise criminal act. The opinions of experts about the "mental state" of defendants ought to be inadmissible in court, exactly as the opinions of experts about the "religious state" of defendants are inadmissible. No one ought to be excused of lawbreaking or any other offense on the basis of so-called expert opinion rendered by psychiatric or mental health experts. Excusing a person of responsibility for an otherwise criminal act on the basis of inability to form conscious intent is an act of legal mercy masquerading as an act of medical science. Being merciful or merciless toward lawbreakers is a moral and legal matter, unrelated to the actual or alleged expertise of medical and mental health professionals.

6. In 1798, Americans were confronted with the task of abolishing slavery, peacefully and without violating the rights of others. They refused to face that daunting task and we are still paying the price of their refusal. In 1998, we Americans are faced with the task of abolishing psychiatric slavery, peacefully and without violating the rights of others. We accept that task and are committed to working for its successful resolution. As Americans before us have eventually replaced involuntary servitude (chattel slavery) with contractual relations between employers and employees, we seek to replace involuntary psychiatry (psychiatric slavery) with contractual relations between care givers and clients.

Thomas Szasz, March 1998

APPENDIX ITEM III: *MENTAL HEALTH, UNITED STATES, 2000*

This report is one of a series published by the United States Department of Health and Human Services—Substance Abuse and Mental Health Services Administration (SAMHSA) National Mental Health

Information Center. It is an overview of a myriad of important issues surrounding mental illness and mental health, many of which are addressed in the previous sections of this book. The entire report, edited by Ronald W. Manderscheid and Marilyn J. Henderson, consists of twenty chapters and four appendices covering topics such as insurance parity, statistics, juvenile justice, organized mental health services, and mental health policies. Each chapter is written by professionals in the relevant area of expertise, from a wide variety of associations, universities, and institutions, including the World Health Organization (WHO). The following excerpt is taken from Section 3: "Status of Mental Health Services at the Millennium" in Chapter 7: "Mental Health Policy at the Millennium: Challenges and Opportunities," written by David Mechanic of the Institute for Health, Health Care Policy and Aging Research Rutgers, the State University of New Jersey. Reference citations for this excerpt can be accessed at http://www.mentalhealth.samhsa.gov/publications/allpubs/SMA01-3537/chapter7.asp, and the index for the entire report can be accessed at http://www.mentalhealth.samhsa.gov/publications/allpubs/SMA01-3537/default.asp. The 1998 and 2002 reports, as well as others published by SAMHSA, can be accessed at http://www.mentalhealth.samhsa.gov/publications/publications_browse.asp?ID=137&Topic=Mental+Health+Care+System.

Mental Health, United States, 2000

Background   The past 50 years have been an extraordinary time for mental health. There have been significant improvements in treatment, public attitudes, and services organization, and enormous growth in mental health insurance coverage, treatment resources, episodes of care, and research of all kinds (Mechanic, 1999). Systems of care have been transformed from largely psychotherapy for the affluent and custodial institutional care for all others to a range of outpatient services, inpatient care in various settings, residential care, and housing alternatives. Mental health care provision, once almost exclusively an activity of State government or fee-for-service private practice, has become an integrated component of health care funded through private and public insurance programs and grants, and appropriations from State, Federal, and local government. State governments that ran most mental health facilities have now substantially reduced their direct role and increasingly are purchasers of care provided by private sector organizations and professionals.

The change now transforming mental health care is the rapid introduction and growth of managed behavioral health care and the numerous ways it is shaping the provision of mental health services and the work of mental health professionals. Managed behavioral health care is very much a work in progress and its ultimate outcomes remain unclear. It offers considerable potential to better organize and rationalize services, and bring to them a more evidence-based culture, but it also presents risks, threatening innovation and appropriate provision of care. These risks seem particularly large for persons with severe and persistent mental illnesses who are more difficult to treat and who may lose ground with the "democratization of care" that occurs under managed behavioral health care (Mechanic & McAlpine, 1999).

In beginning a new century, it is important to look back at both the gains and the unanticipated consequences of mental health policy, and the implications they have for what lies ahead. Health organization and policy never arise anew. They evolve from prior culture and understandings, health care arrangements, health professional organizations, and political and economic processes. Mental health has been shaped as much by cultural changes and major social policies designed with other populations in mind as by the efforts of persons working in the mental health field itself. These changes and policies include the broader economic, political, and legal ideologies and influences that supported deinstitutionalization of persons with mental illness and those with other types of disabilities; the introduction of major national health insurance programs such as Medicaid and Medicare, which stimulated the development of new facilities, professionals, and incentives; and Social Security Disability Insurance and Supplemental Security Income (SSI), which facilitated community residence and subsistence. In the past several decades, there were advances in drugs and other technologies, in ways of managing patients within community programs, and in increased consumer involvement and public acceptance. Taking advantage of these changes, however, requires an appropriate institutional framework for financing, organization, and delivery, which are highly dependent on macro social policy.

As we proceed into a new century, mental health policy and services remain areas with considerable controversy. There have been significant research advances and improvements in treatment, but experts continue to disagree on the nature of mental illness and what dysfunctions are diseases in a medical sense and which are extensions of normal distress. The longstanding debate on the extent to which mental disorders are discrete categorical conditions or part of a broad continuum also persists. Underlying differences in perspective then link to philosophical and public policy questions such as the degree to which persons with mental disorders should be held responsible for their behavior and the tradeoffs between coercion and liberty in decisions about involuntary treatment. These perspectives also affect broader public reactions such as stigmatization and discrimination against persons with mental illness and the willingness of the public to support the necessary investments to close the gaps between unmet need and treatment.

This chapter is organized around six areas: deinstitutionalization; improved treatment technologies; the larger societal context and debates concerning parity; the legal context; managed behavioral health care; and the growth of consumer involvement. In each case, tensions are evident in seeking the appropriate balance among contending interests, philosophies, and research perspectives. For each major point, there are counterpoints reflecting the continuing struggle over defining the appropriate domains of mental disorder and the distribution of responsibilities among the Federal Government, State and local governments, the nonprofit and private sectors, the helping professions, and persons with mental illness and their families.

Deinstitutionalization   The most enduring change in the post–World War II period has been the deinstitutionalization of persons with mental illness (Grob, 1994), a trend now continuing under managed care arrangements (Mechanic, 1998a). Many factors contributed to this movement including social ideologies, the introduction of new drugs, changing social attitudes toward persons with mental illness and toward institutional care, the desire to reduce State government expenditures, litigation on behalf of persons with mental illness, and public welfare programs that made it possible to house and provide income support and other services to clients with disabilities in the community (Mechanic, 1999). Managed care maintains the deinstitutionalization trend, continuing to reduce inpatient care. It is potentially an instrument to better allocate care; but, in managing costs, it also reduces expenditures for purchasers and allows profits for private companies and their stockholders, thus reducing the funding available for direct service provision.

Public mental hospitals have been reduced or downsized from 560,000 resident patients in 1955 to fewer than 60,000 clients today, despite sizable population growth. Most acute inpatient care is now in general hospitals; and although case-mix and comorbidity are more complex, average length of stay has fallen steadily to less than 10 days, and continues to fall. In the period 1988 to 1994, some 12.5 million days were reduced in mental hospital care with only small compensation in days of care in the general hospital sector (Mechanic, McAlpine, & Olfson, 1998). The introduction of managed care in the private sector has reduced expenditures of some large corporate purchasers by as much as 30–40 percent, with most of these reductions achieved by large reductions in average length of stay (Feldman, 1998; Mechanic & McAlpine, 1999).

There is much debate on the consequences of such changes with allegations that care has significantly deteriorated, that patients are being discharged from hospitals "quicker and sicker," and that persons floridly ill are discharged to homelessness, neglect, victimization, and violent encounters (Isaac & Armat, 1990). Problems in care are common and are attributable to the deficiency of community services and the difficult task of providing the supervision and care available in hospitals, particularly to uncooperative clients, in dispersed settings in the community. Undesirable outcomes are inevitable when supervision is relaxed for high-risk patient populations. There are many deficiencies in access to and the comprehensiveness of community care, but allegations concerning the failures of deinstitutionalization ignore the large social and human costs of alternative policies (Mechanic, 1999). The traditional custodial mental hospital ruined many lives. But many communities, even now, have yet to develop the networks of community services essential to an effective system of deinstitutionalized care. Nevertheless, the evidence is overwhelming that most clients are immeasurably better off in the deinstitutionalized care system than they ever could be in mental hospitals. It remains less clear, however, whether reduced hospitalization has been too extensive and is now introducing unacceptable risks to persons with complex mental health needs.

One significant criticism of the extent of deinstitutionalization is that it has contributed to "criminalization" of persons with mental illness. The extent of such criminalization is difficult to assess because of increased inclusion of deviant behavior within psychiatric categories and particularly the inclusion of substance abuse and antisocial behavior. Arrests commonly involve such behavior (Hiday, 1999). The jail and prison population has grown substantially and now includes many persons who have *Diagnostic and Statistical Manual* (DSM) disorders, but it is difficult to determine how large a change this is from prior periods when such disorders were not recognized or defined as such. Nevertheless, the freedom of community life, the fragmentation of service systems, easy availability and use of substances, and the unavailability of hospital beds for other than short-term acute care make it inevitable that many persons with serious mental illness in the community will, at some time, face arrest.

A Justice Department study estimated that in midyear 1998, there were more than 280,000 persons with mental illness in jails and prisons, and more than a half million more on probation (Ditton, 1999). Although the methods used to assess and count mental illnesses were crude, the findings suggest the magnitude of the problem. Many of the violations committed for which people were incarcerated occurred under the influence of alcohol and drugs, and persons with substance abuse comorbidities are involved disproportionately in instances of violent behavior (Steadman et al., 1998). The substantially increased pattern of substance use and abuse associated with severe mental illness in the community poses serious treatment and management problems. Also, persons with mental illness in prisons have more difficulty with prison life and are more likely to get into fights and commit other rule violations (Ditton, 1999).

Some persons with mental illness have committed serious and violent crimes and require secure detention. But many are in jails and prisons by virtue of community neglect and lack of appropriate treatment. Others have repeatedly committed nuisance offenses and are jailed only for short periods, sometimes as "compassionate arrests" to get them off the streets and out of dangerous situations. Nevertheless, the criminalization of their behavior reinforces stigmatization that is already a barrier to community support and care, and complicates relationships with family, caretakers, and the community.

As we begin a new century, the decriminalization of mental illness and provision of a safe and appropriate environment for those who must remain in detention will have to be addressed more intensively. Avoiding criminalization will require aggressive and effective community care services and diversion programs that appropriately reroute patients into mental health systems of care. Improved mental health services in jails and prisons also are needed. Collaboration between the mental health and criminal justice systems always has been difficult and the complications of managed care contracting will not make it easier. Different cultures and priorities impose barriers to effective communication and collaboration.

The fundamental challenge is to fulfill the promises of deinstitutionalization policies faithfully by developing well-organized and balanced systems of community care with a broad spectrum of services and clear focus of responsibility and accountability. Such services must include assertive case management; sophisticated medication management; attention to housing, work, and needed social supports; substance abuse education and treatment; and many more. After several decades, we are finally seeing more States and localities developing assertive community treatment teams for those with more serious and persistent conditions. Managed behavioral health care was believed to have the incentives to create more balanced systems of care within a deinstitutionalized system, but this potential is yet to be demonstrated (Mechanic, 1998b; Mechanic & McAlpine, 1999).

Improving Treatment Technologies   A second major change in the later decades of the past century was the introduction of new approaches to investigate the scientific bases of mental illness and the application of tools from molecular biology, genetics, behavioral science, epidemiology, and health services research (U.S. Department of Health and Human Services, 1999). New imaging technologies have made it possible to directly track changes in the brain and to potentially use such observations for specific targeting of drugs. Although the payoffs from this sophisticated scientific infrastructure development are yet to be realized, the scientific advances set the stage for substantially improved understanding and treatment in the new century.

The scientific approach to mental illness has become more sophisticated and rigorous and the standards for evidence have been elevated. After many decades of psychoanalytic dominance and facile theorizing, research models and standards for evidence have tightened significantly. Psychiatry as a profession has moved closer to medicine, investigation has accelerated on the biological dimensions of psychiatric disorders, and research collaboration among disciplines in psychiatry and the behavioral sciences is more common. Randomized controlled trials have become the gold standard in evaluating interventions and there is a greater focus on evidence-based practice.

There has also been growing realization that research results obtained under highly controlled conditions in research centers with carefully selected patients cannot necessarily be generalized to the unwieldy patterns of practice in the community. There now is increased attention to the gap between efficacy studies and effectiveness of practice. Moreover, health services research studies show significant failures to provide the treatments that are best supported by research evidence (Lehman & Steinwachs, 1998; Wells, Sturm, Sherbourne, & Meredith, 1996), and it is inevitable that overcoming barriers and developing strategies for dissemination and implementation will be high on our agenda in the coming decades.

Although we have yet to have fundamental advances in drug therapy, the medications now available for treatment of schizophrenia, depression, and other major mental illnesses have improved. Newer drugs such as selective serotonin reuptake inhibitors (SSRIs) and atypical antipsychotics appear generally to be no more efficacious than earlier medications, but they have fewer side effects and are tolerated more easily, facilitating medication adherence and improved outcomes. The unwillingness of many persons with serious mental illness to continue on their medications constitutes one of the most serious obstacles to effective management and will continue to be a major focus of attention in treatment and research. The availability of a larger range of medications also facilitates treatment because patients have atypical and unpredictable responses to medications, and more options increases the probability of identifying compatible treatments. In schizophrenia, patients unresponsive to other drugs often respond remarkably well to clozapine, which has become an important backup treatment for patients who fail on the more commonly used medications. Although the thrust of pharmaceutical development and marketing has been on the specificity of drug action, there is ample evidence that many of the common medications affect a range of seemingly different disorders (Healy, 1997).

Mental health services research also has demonstrated the advantages of a variety of psychosocial management approaches from assertive community treatment to family psycho-education (Lehman & Steinwachs, 1998). These social technologies have been more difficult to disseminate than new medications, and services studies show that most patients who can benefit still do not receive such treatment (Lehman & Steinwachs, 1998; Young, Sullivan, Burnam, & Brook, 1998). Nevertheless, there has been growing appreciation of the importance of these management approaches and slow but increasing adoption. Assertive community treatment is accepted widely as the best available approach for managing severe and persistent illness in the community. We can anticipate more energy devoted to implementation and further study of the type and intensity of management that best fits varying client populations.

As we begin a new century, our hopes and expectations are high, but our understanding of the major mental illnesses is still limited. Our tools and approaches for studying these problems are improved, but history teaches us that it is easy to make claims of being on the threshold (Grob, 1998). A certain modesty is needed, as well as a willingness to be open to new conceptualizations, theories, methods, and approaches. The DSM is an important example. Developed as a descriptive convenience to help standardize scientific work and practice and to improve communication, DSM has been reified by many practitioners and decisionmakers in ways that are not constructive. Inconsistent with its own conceptual view of mental illness, and probably greatly overinclusive (Regier et al., 1998; Wakefield 1997, 1996), DSM is no more than a convenient instrument and should not be used as a standard to limit research on alternative approaches. It introduces and reinforces conceptions of greater specificity of mental disorders than can be validated empirically (Healy, 1997). The profusion of diagnostic entities probably partly explains the degree of comorbidity reported in most studies.

Views of mental illness and mental health policy have cycled widely over the years between biological and social conceptions, often exaggerated at both extremes. This cycling occasionally is useful as a strategy because it helps move a particular line of research forward. However, research on mental illness is served poorly by disciplinary parochialism. Most of the mental illnesses have to be understood in a multicausal context requiring consideration of biology, social structures, human development, and social processes. Science policy in the future should enable such cross-disciplinary fertilization and cooperation.

Given the many uncertainties that continue to characterize treatment of mental disorders, there is concern with the present focus on biological aspects and the preference of managed care for medication treatments over psychotherapy, counseling, or other modalities. Such direct approaches as interpersonal psychotherapy and rehabilitation approaches remain important as alternative treatments or as adjuncts to medication. They often are fundamental to facilitating greater personal comfort, improved social function, and higher quality of life.

Mental Illness and Mental Health Policy in a Societal Context   The prevalence of mental illness varies substantially among nations and among various social and cultural groups within countries, regions, and communities (Dohrenwend et al., 1992; Weissman et al., 1996). The occurrence of some mental illnesses, such as schizophrenia, is more invariant than most, but even rates of schizophrenia will vary substantially among some subgroups (Bhugra et al., 1997; Harrison et al., 1997). Some of the environmental contributors to some mental illnesses may include nutrition, birth practices, infections, and epidemics; but the causal factors and how they interact with genetic and other biological risk factors remain unknown. Major depression and substance abuse, two of the most common mental disorders, are very much influenced by social and cultural factors, and factors in individuals' lives and relationships (Brown & Harris, 1978; Horwitz & Scheid, 1999).

Socioeconomic status has one of the strongest associations with the prevalence of mental disorders (Dohrenwend et al., 1992; Eaton & Muntaner, 1999) as well as many physical conditions, but the causal pathways involved are complex, multidimensional, and incompletely understood (Amick, Levine, Tarlov, & Walsh, 1995; Dohrenwend et al., 1992; Link & Phelan, 1995; Wilkinson, 1996). Nevertheless, it is reasonably clear that social structures make their mark on the occurrence of psychiatric morbidity through class, culture, and gender. Although the relationship between social structure and mental illness has been observed for

100 years or more, there is now renewed interest in how social structures might be modified to reduce disability and improve health (Benzeval, Judge, & Whitehead, 1995). Although there is much research on contributory factors such as helplessness, fatalism, social support, coping, and the like (Horwitz & Scheid, 1999), it remains uncertain how such understanding can be translated usefully into efforts to improve mental health, especially in the case of the major mental illnesses. Yet, there are many good research leads that require further development (Mrazek & Haggerty, 1994).

The Uninsured, Undertreatment, and Unmet Need

More apparent is the continuing evidence that most persons with mental illness remain untreated (Kessler et al., 1994; McAlpine & Mechanic, 2000), that those who are treated often receive inappropriate and incorrect treatment (Wells et al., 1996; Lehman & Steinwachs, 1998), and that mental disorders remain highly stigmatized and neglected. Social policies have a major role in making treatment available. Persons with serious and persistent mental illness remain perhaps the most disadvantaged and neglected group in our society and suffer from the failures of American health care policy. The United States remains the only major nation in the world without universal health insurance. In the past decade, despite a growing and highly successful economy, the number of uninsured persons has grown (Kronick & Gilmer, 1999). Persons with serious mental illness are disproportionately uninsured (McAlpine & Mechanic, 2000). Many others with health insurance have only very limited coverage for mental health and substance abuse services, which typically are not available on the same basis as other types of care and limited by more deductibles, coinsurance, and caps (Buck, Teich, Umland, & Stein, 1999; Mechanic & McAlpine, 1999).

The Parity Issue

In recent years there has been growing interest in parity of mental health with other medical services. Legislative efforts have been made at both State and Federal levels, but the concept of parity varies from one context to another and the level of legislative intervention varies a great deal as well. The underlying idea of parity is that the same range and comprehensiveness of insurance benefits available for other illnesses should apply as well to persons with mental illness and substance abuse problems. There is a growing political constituency for parity among influential consumer groups and some politicians, and we are likely to see continuing efforts in the future. A major concern to policy-makers has been the cost of parity, since research indicates that some mental health services (particularly psychotherapy) are more responsive to insurance coverage than other types of medical services (Frank & McGuire, 1986; McGuire, 1981). Parity in a managed care context is more palatable because cost can be held readily in check through managed care strategies and the additional premium costs required for more complete mental health coverage appear to be modest (Goldman, McCulloch, & Sturm, 1998; Sturm, 1997). Moreover, some influential consumer groups like the National Alliance for the Mentally Ill (NAMI) would restrict the application of parity to the major mental illnesses, conditions they refer to as diseases of the brain.

Nevertheless, there are serious issues with the application of the parity concept, particularly as it affects persons with serious and persistent mental illness, and numerous issues remain unresolved. First, managed care purports to provide "all necessary services" (Mechanic, 1998a), but many of the services required by persons with serious mental illness are excluded from "medical necessity" definitions. Indeed, more than half the expenditures required for persons in the community with severe mental illness are usually not covered by conventional health insurance (Hollingsworth & Sweeney, 1997). Thus, benefit designs cannot depend on vague definitions of medical necessity and need to be clearly specified. This may involve services not typically problematic in the treatment of persons with physical illness, such as assistance in becoming adequately housed. It should be noted, however, that many of these sociomedical services become more commonly needed with population aging and the management of chronic disease and disability.

Second, because standards of mental health care are less clear than for surgical and medical treatment, such care seems to be managed in a more rigorous way with much larger reductions of treatment requested by physicians (Mechanic & McAlpine, 1999; Wickizer & Lessler, 1998). Moreover, there is evidence that while the management process seems to provide a nominal primary health service to more people than typically found in fee-for-service practice, those with the greatest need and disadvantage receive less intense services. Decision processes seem not sufficiently sensitive to the seriousness and complexity of illness, and patients with the most severe illnesses appear to do less well under present management arrangements as compared to fee-for-service practice (Mechanic, 1998b, 1999). Inclusion of parity for mental health services within a "medical necessity" definition has no real meaning if services are not reasonably accessible, appropriate, and of high quality (Mechanic & McAlpine, 1999). There is still a great deal to learn about these management processes and their relationship to quality of care. Good evidence on the effects of managed care on the severely and persistently ill population is difficult to obtain because varied outcomes have to be assessed over reasonably long periods and few studies do this.

The Difficulty of Establishing Boundaries for Mental Health Coverage

Many policymakers, while sympathetic to the idea that persons with mental illness should have access to treatment comparable to those with other types of disorders, worry about opening the flood-gates to increased utilization and costs. The appeal of managed care and the idea of using a "medical necessity" definition is that tight controls are in place to manage potential overutilization. We now have a large number of clinicians from many disciplines and professions prepared to offer reimbursed services for persons with mental illness. It is well established that a major determinant of utilization and costs is the supply of reimbursable services available and, thus, without some form of gatekeeping, utilization could expand in irrational and costly ways. There are a number of alternative solutions. One form of control is to have different levels of cost-sharing depending on the service and the extent of moral hazard. Thus, services like diagnostic assessment, medication management, and inpatient care may have lower cost-sharing than psychotherapy, a service that often is attractive to persons with lesser disorders, for existential and self-realization reasons. This approach is unpopular with such professions as psychology and social work, which provide much of the psychotherapy.

A common approach, based on the notion that persons with more severe conditions should receive priority, is to restrict the definition of conditions covered by the parity concept to several of the major mental disorders such as schizophrenia, major depression, and bipolar disorders. These are typically referred to by proponents as "diseases of the brain" and distinguished from other disorders which presumably are not. This distinction, while practical, may be both too inclusive and too exclusive. It is unclear that all of the more serious disorders usually suggested for coverage are "disease of the brain" except in the trivial sense that all behavior is mediated by the brain. Nor is it evident that some seemingly less serious conditions are not. Many conditions that would be excluded under these suggested definitions are painful and seriously interfere with function. Many may, indeed, offer opportunities for improved outcomes that are comparable or better than outcomes achieved in the case of the most serious mental illnesses (Mrazek & Haggerty, 1994). As we look toward a fairer system of health insurance, we require the application of tools that allow us to assess the cost-effectiveness of alternative interventions, while remaining sensitive to other community values as well (Ubel, 2000).

The Legal Context of Mental Health Services   In the 1970's, legal activists in mental health almost "made a revolution" (Appelbaum, 1994) around a range of issues including right to treatment, right to refuse treatment, involuntary commitment, and least restrictive alternatives, among others. After a flurry of turmoil, disputes abated and these contentious matters reached a certain equilibrium. A variety of new legal issues of large import are now emerging and are likely to have an important impact on future mental health services.

One new potential instrument is the Americans with Disabilities Act (ADA) and the U.S. Supreme Court decision in *Olmstead* vs. *L. C.* which required the State of Georgia to provide community care to persons with mental illnesses and mental retardation who could function in such less restrictive settings without placing an undue burden on the State or requiring that the State establish a particular type of program. The decision was sufficiently qualified to be uncertain about its ultimate reach, but the ADA adds an additional instrument through which persons with mental illness and their advocates can challenge arrangements and programs that limit their opportunity for fuller community participation. Lawyers representing persons with mental illness also are using ADA to challenge discrimination in health insurance (Moss, Ullman, Starrett, Burris, & Johnsen, 1999).

The litigation of earlier decades was focused on increasing the rights of persons with mental illness and reducing coercive controls. Current legal approaches, in contrast, are more focused on developing mechanisms that support deinstitutionalization by imposing more controls on living in the community. Outpatient commitment or other conditions for remaining in the community are more common today, despite difficult legal dilemmas, as a way of inducing patients who are at risk to maintain contact with treatment programs and to take their medications (Torrey & Kaplan, 1995). Here, the threat of hospitalization may be a significant deterrent to noncooperation, although the legal basis for imposing limits on freedom in the community is more debatable and contested. A recent study of outpatient commitment in New York found that outpatient commitment had some success in reducing subsequent hospital readmissions, but the effects were explained by the intensity of service provision (Swartz et al., 1999). The effects, thus, came not from the legal intervention itself but from the fact that the intervention was linked to providing more services to clients. The underlying issue is the quality and intensity of the services available to clients in the community.

The Challenges of Managed Behavioral Health Care

About three-quarters of Americans with health insurance are now under some form of managed behavioral health program. Although there are complaints about managed behavioral health care, particularly with respect to access to specialty services, and intensity of care, the industry has demonstrated its capacity to reduce private sector costs considerably without much evidence of impairing care (Mechanic, 1999). One of the advantages of behavioral health care carve-out arrangements is that they tend to give more people access to at least some specialty mental health services than occurs under the fee-for-service system. Intensity of care is much reduced, however, particularly regarding inpatient services and extensive psychotherapy (Mechanic, 1998b; Mechanic & McAlpine, 1999).

A significant limitation of carve-outs is the lack of coordination between mental health and substance abuse services, and other medical services. Even mental health and substance abuse may be separately carved out with prescriptions involving still another carve-out. The fragmentation of care and boundary problems that occur can be substantial; but, thus far, there is little evidence that integrated care is a high priority. The ideal of integrated care is widely endorsed, but, with current pressures on clinicians, the realities of high-quality integrated care are challenging. Despite several decades of effort in attempting to make primary care clinicians more receptive to and skilled at providing mental health services, their performance in recognizing and treating psychiatric illness remains limited (Mechanic, 1997; Wells et al., 1996). Carve-outs, whatever their limitations, organize providers of care who are interested in behavioral health problems and experienced in managing them.

One significant advantage of managed behavioral health care is the opportunity to introduce practice standards and guidelines in a systematic way. Studies of quality care repeatedly indicate poor performance as measured by the scientific evidence about appropriate treatment of even such major conditions as schizophrenia and major depression. Managed behavioral health care has the potential to bring practice more in line with the evidence base. If managed behavioral health care was working successfully, we would expect a close relationship between intensity of care and severity of illness and disability, and evidence of substitution of care when more intensive treatments are reduced. Unfortunately, there is little evidence in support of these expectations (Mechanic & McAlpine, 1999).

The role of managed behavioral health care for populations of those more severely and persistently ill is problematic and uncertain in the future. The idea of managing care is hardly new for this population—it typically has been served by public programs with scarce resources and the need to make allocations carefully. Over several decades, mental health professionals and administrators in the public sector in many States developed a broad community support structure that fit the wide range of needs of persons with serious mental illnesses in the community. To the extent that States shift this responsibility to private managed care companies, which have little experience managing the needs of such highly disadvantaged populations, the outcomes become more uncertain. States have had varying experiences with managed care for persons with serious mental illness; but it is not clear that the private sector has an appropriate infrastructure in place for such care and, if it does, whether it can profit from providing such management. There are some indications that managed behavioral health care companies are backing off public contracts for the psychiatrically disabled population, and States, too, are being cautious.

Managed care is a work in progress, and patterns of management change fairly quickly. Thus, it is difficult to know how this sector will evolve, what adaptations it will make as it gains experience, or whether it will survive in its present forms. Managed care in the general medical sphere has been highly adaptive in response to public criticism, and has increased access to specialty care and made other changes consistent with consumer concerns. It has sought to reduce tensions resulting from utilization management by shifting risk to provider groups so that utilization review could be relaxed. There has been little such transfer of risk in behavioral health and little confidence that provider groups would know how to manage such risk. Thus, almost all reductions of cost have come from reduced inpatient care and negotiated reductions in rates. With increased competition, capitation payments have been driven to levels that make one skeptical that an appropriate pattern of care can be maintained, particularly after administrative costs and profits are extracted from the system of care.

The Growth of Consumer Involvement

One of the remarkable changes in mental health services has been the increasing involvement of consumer groups that play an important advocacy and political role, and that have developed a wide range of self-help and informal care services (Kaufmann, 1999). Many of the consumer services are consumer-run or administered by professionals committed to an empowerment philosophy that regards consumers as members rather than clients. These various groups may have different philosophies and ideologies, view mental health differently, have different treatment preferences, and often compete in their advocacy. Both the Federal and State governments have worked with these advocacy and consumer groups and have supported their development. The informal and self-help sectors are a very significant component of the system of mental health services (Kessler et al., 1999).

The National Mental Health Association (NMHA) dates back to Clifford Beers and the mental hygiene movement early in the century. NAMI—an organization less than 25 years old—has also become a highly influential mental health advocacy group. NAMI's membership of about 210,000 includes persons with mental illness and their family members. The organization has built a powerful State and Federal constituency that lobbies extensively; partners with professionals, researchers, and advocates; carries out extensive communications and educational programs; and sponsors its own research program. While NAMI's membership is diverse, the organization strongly endorses a focus on the most serious mental disorders. NAMI's political agenda is to support biomedical and health services research funding, parity in health care coverage, and improved care for persons with mental illness. NAMI has formed strategic alliances with members of Congress and the Executive branch and with many key policymakers in the States. As a federation of local organizations, NAMI provides support to its local AMIs who in many States are quite effective in promoting legislative initiatives.

NAMI is sometimes at odds with other mental health organizations and groups that favor different priorities. Although NAMI, at times, has been highly critical of mental health professionals, it opposes groups who reject the idea of mental illnesses as diseases and who reject medication. NAMI supports the use of civil commitment and more forceful interventions in opposition to liberty advocates. NAMI also sometimes comes into conflict with NMHA on the range of conditions to be included in mental health legislation and on the priority the NMHA gives to preventive efforts and public education. In the inevitable conflicts between persons with mental illnesses and their families, NAMI generally advocates for families and for means of reducing their burden in caring for a relative with mental illness.

The empowerment philosophy advocated by clubhouses such as Foundation House and by consumer-administered self-help programs and drop-in centers also sometimes comes into conflict with NAMI philosophy. There is no single viewpoint that pervades these programs, and clubhouses modeled after Fountain House may be quite different from one another or consumer-run services. But in some instances members adopt an antipsychiatry and antimedication view. They also commonly side with members in conflict with families. We know little definitively about the value of mental health consumer-run services, but both theory and research suggest that empowerment can be a powerful influence on how clients view themselves and their quality of life (Rosenfield, 1992).

The best known of all self-help efforts is Alcoholics Anonymous (AA) and its 12-step program. Twelve-step programs are now widely used in formal treatment settings as well as by community groups. With the increasing use of alcohol and drugs, "double trouble" groups appear to be growing. They offer persons with mental illness a more supportive environment for maintaining their medications than traditional AA groups. One significant problem in behavioral health advocacy is the conflict among groups advocating for attention for different disorders such as mental illness, alcoholism, substance use disorder, and developmental disabilities. The lack of more united advocacy limits mental health efforts relative to other important disease advocacy organizations.

A New Century

Much is uncertain about the future of mental health services. A few observations are quite firm, however. First, although there is much wishful thinking and rhetoric about advances, there remains a great deal we do not know. Many mental disorders remain intractable, and treatment is still often on a hit-or-miss basis. How soon advances in neuroscience and molecular genetics will bring new and more effective treatments remains uncertain. Second, there is considerable evidence that the treatments we do have are not well distributed because of insurance limitations, public stigma, lack of patient choice, and professional ignorance. The failure to use our existing science base and research evidence must be high on the agenda as we begin this new century. The evidence is that we do much better at disseminating new drug treatments than behavioral programs, but even in the drug area, current practice is seriously deficient.

Again, it is important to understand that the future of mental health treatment is as likely to depend on policy decisions outside the mental health sector as within it. Perhaps most important is whether our Nation can move to a system of universal access to care and whether the benefit design covers those services that we know are invaluable for persons with serious mental disorders. Such community care will also depend on the strength of public social supports such as those dealing with income maintenance, housing, work rehabilitation, and the like. It will also depend on community attitudes, feelings of safety, and levels of tolerance.

In the past several decades, American society has changed dramatically in its view of persons with disabilities. These individuals now participate in all aspects of community life. The passage and implementation of the ADA reinforce these changes and break new ground for further advances for full participation. Prominent individuals who have struggled with mental illnesses, including authors, politicians, celebrities, sports figures, and others, are now more likely to publicly acknowledge and discuss what were previously deeply held secrets. Many more people are now willing to seek treatment, and mental health care is more respectable among general physicians. Nevertheless, mental illness remains stigmatized and discrediting, and public perceptions still remain punitive relative to other disabling conditions. This is particularly true of persons with psychoses and those with substance abuse disorders. In the latter case, provision of treatment is particularly inadequate, with long waiting lists for access to treatment and punitive official policies. Persons with substance disorders are commonly seen as the "undeserving sick" in the public eye (Mechanic, 1999).

Study of history tells us that social policy does not progress in a linear fashion and often moves in cycles of advance and retrogression. Thus, it is impossible to foresee how the tensions relating to the identification and treatment of persons with mental illness may play out in the future. Few observers anticipated that 40 years after implementing an ideological victory to replace custodial mental health care with a community public health approach, we would have to address the problem of hundreds of thousands of persons with mental illness in jails, in prisons, or on probation and the large numbers of homeless persons with mental illness seen on the streets of all our large cities. Yet, the vast majority of persons with mental illnesses today lead better lives, get more effective treatment, and are less stigmatized than in the past. Effective treatment of mental illness in future decades will depend on advances in knowledge and technology, and on the social and political factors that affect social policies in general and mental health policies in particular.

APPENDIX ITEM IV: A LETTER BY JEFFREY A. SCHALER, PH.D.

Schaler is adjunct professor, Department of Justice, Law, and Society, American University, Washington, D.C. This letter is in response to an opinion column written by Morton S. Rapp, psychiatrist at Scarborough Hospital, Toronto, Ontario. Both were published in the *Medical Post* and can be accessed on at http://www.schaler.net/hasszaszlearned.html.

The following letter to the editor was published in the June 6, 1995, issue of *The Medical Post* (Vol. 31, No. 22), page 12. Reprinted with permission by J. A. Schaler, Ph.D. and www.szasz.com.

Why Single Out Dr. Szasz for His Views?

To the Editor: Morton Rapp attacks Thomas Szasz's character, not his ideas, in his opinion piece, "Has Dr. Szasz Learned Anything over the Years?" (The Medical Post, March 21).

Argument ad hominem appeals to feelings rather than intellect and, according to [Eugene] Ehrlich, "is considered a logical fallacy, in that such an argument fails to prove a point by failing to address it."

Dr. Rapp refuses to address the matter at hand—the myth of mental illness and its relation to civil commitment.

That aside, Dr. Rapp claims "a landmark case of alleged psychiatric negligence has recently been settled in the United States." How can "alleged" negligence be a "landmark case"?

Surely Dr. Rapp knows that an accusation of wrongdoing does not constitute guilt. There was no finding of negligence in the civil lawsuit filed against Dr. Szasz.

Cynically, Dr. Rapp asks why Dr. Szasz continues to practise psychiatry since he "has been preaching . . . the doctrine that there is no such thing as mental illness": Practising psychiatry is not contingent upon believing in the existence of mental illness.

Is there an oath regarding belief in "mental illness" that one must now take to belong in the church of psychiatry? Many psychiatrists practice psychotherapy. Their clients find the conversation called psychotherapy useful. Believing in "mental illness" has nothing to do with it!

Moreover, if Dr. Rapp would take time to read Dr. Szasz's voluminous works he'd discover that Szasz has always differentiated between institutional and contractual psychiatry.

Dr. Rapp states that the psychiatrist who engaged in a contractual relationship with Dr. Szasz and later committed suicide was "suffering from bipolar affective disorder ('manic-depressive psychosis')." That diagnosis is based on a newspaper account of the deceased. That's an unethical way to present an allegedly definitive diagnosis.

Finally, Dr. Rapp confuses explanations for behavioral events with the events themselves, a common mistake.

Schizophrenia is a label used to explain abnormal behavior, usually characterized by false claims and self-reported imaginings, e.g., hallucination.

Schizophrenia is not an event—it is one explanation for an event. Biological explanations for abnormal behavior are not the events Dr. Rapp claims as "mental illness." That's why mental illness is not listed in standard textbooks on pathology.

Descriptions of an explanation for mental illness do not meet the nosological criteria for disease classification.

Why does Dr. Rapp rail against Dr. Szasz when pathologists, clearly experts on disease, do not consider mental illness a real disease too?

Dr. Rapp's vituperation notwithstanding, Dr. Szasz is clearly one of the most important writers and thinkers of this century. His ideas will continue to be a thorn in the side of the "therapeutic state" until the power of government no longer fuels the Inquisition of Institutional Psychiatry.

Based on the excitement my students consistently express about Dr. Szasz's work, I suspect that day is not far off.

Reproduced with permission by J. A. Schaler, Ph.D. and www.szasz.com.

In reply to the following:

From *The Medical Post*, a publication for the Canadian medical profession, March 21, 1995, page 12, opinion column entitled "I say, I say":

Has Dr. Szasz Learned Anything over the Years?

by Morton S. Rapp

A landmark case of alleged psychiatric negligence has recently been settled in the United States, and considering that it contains all those elements which make for a media spectacle, it is amazing this case has been neglected by the press.

The defendant was Dr. Thomas Szasz, 74, psychiatric renegade, who has been preaching for the last 40 years, in books, lectures and public forums, the doctrine that there is no such thing as mental illness. (Why he then continued to practise psychiatry is something for him to explain.)

The plaintiff was the estate of a psychiatrist-patient suffering from bipolar affective disorder ("manic-depressive psychosis") who consulted Dr. Szasz after being first treated by a more traditional physician.

The issue is that the patient wasn't taking his lithium during treatment with Dr. Szasz, presumably became depressed, and committed suicide.

The legal settlement included an agreement that neither side would "voluntarily seek publicity" in the matter, so it is difficult to determine, for example, whether the patient stopped his lithium and then sought out Dr. Szasz's help or whether Dr. Szasz encouraged the patient.

The only thing that's clear is Dr. Szasz paid $650,000 US to the family of the deceased in settlement.

Dr. Szasz did not begin his professional career as an iconoclast. Some of his early work dealt with, for example, some very sophisticated theoretical considerations about pain.

However, few people have paid much attention to his early work. Dr. Szasz became widely known as a result of publishing a series of books which described a way of looking at psychiatry, psychiatric patients, and psychiatric treatment and practice in a manner which can only be called conspiratorial and paranoid.

To Dr. Szasz, the entire psychiatric apparatus served the function of isolating dissidents from mainstream society, using "mental health laws" to strip patients of their right, and employing instruments of torture (e.g. electroconvulsive therapy) disguised as "helpful treatments."

He even claimed the entire concept of mental illness was a convenient fiction enabling white-coated agents of society to carry out this function.

His conception of American psychiatry in the 1950s did not differ radically from the historically proven abusive system then existing in the Soviet Union, where 5% of psychiatric facilities were indeed used for the purpose of containing, discrediting and often destroying political opponents.

Of course, if the concept of "mental illness" is to be denied, then the actions of "patients" somehow have to be explained in terms other than their suffering from "schizophrenia" or "bipolar disorder."

It became a little difficult to explain why the "oppressed dissidents" occupying the psychiatric asylums of the U.S. didn't stop acting that way when released, or why they so closely resembled their untreated and neglected brethren in other countries. But somehow Dr. Szasz was able to convince himself of the continued rightness of his beliefs.

It is often say [*sic*] by critics with more forgiveness than this writer that while Dr. Szasz's essential ideas were disastrously wrong (or, in words attributed to Nobel winner Edelman, "so bad they are not even wrong"), he nevertheless uncovered and helped to curtail certain specific excesses and injustices in the system.

I don't think this is true. Dr. Szasz was against electroconvulsive therapy for the usual reasons, but ECT disappeared not because of his rhetoric, but because it could be replaced by antidepressant and antipsychotic drugs, so it was no longer the only psychiatric modality that actually worked.

Similarly, the much more narrow definition of which psychiatric patients could be detained against their will resulted from two factors unrelated to Dr. Szasz's pronouncements.

First, human rights were in ascendancy. Second, the newer drug treatments were producing a larger population of mentally ill who could safely reside outside hospitals.

Having said all this, however, an admission must be made that in the 1960s, when Dr. Szasz's books were getting close attention both from fellow anti-psychiatrists and also from bewildered and defensive members of "the establishment," there was one fact that made his ideas sustainable.

That was that we knew absolutely nothing about brain pathology, neurohormones or the biological relationships among thinking, feeling and behavior.

But this has changed. We have overwhelming evidence of the genetic transmission of at least the propensity to become mentally ill. We have machines that can register metabolic differences in the brains of people with schizophrenia and people without it.

We have machines that can differentiate when one is thinking about a tomato, and when one is thinking about slicing a tomato. And we have drugs which take advantage of our still primitive, but at least extant, knowledge of brain chemistry, to effect symptomatic cures of diseases once thought incurable, including resistant schizophrenia.

Not all anti-psychiatrists of the past clung so tenaciously to their ideas.

For example, Dr. R. D. Laing, a British psychiatrist and darling of the '60s counterculture, originally declared that schizophrenia was not a disease, but a response of a sane person to an insane set of social controls, administered by the patient's parents.

However, in response to the growing biological science of mental disorders, he recanted this belief shortly before his death, though not in time to undo so much human misery he caused with his mistaken pronouncements.

Dr. Thomas Szasz, as far as one can tell at a distance, seems not to have incorporated the enormous knowledge base about the brain and behavior accumulating at an exponential rate since at least the '70s. Like the Bourbons, he seems to have learned nothing and forgotten nothing.

Morton Rapp is a psychiatrist in Willowdale, Ont.

Permission given by Morton S. Rapp, M.D., The Scarborough Hospital, Toronto.

Mental Illness Timeline

Prehistory   Magical orientation. Shamans use rituals and spells to exorcise causative spirits. Trepanation perhaps believed to release the spirit trapped within.

2850 BC   Ancient Egypt: magical origin with a religious dimension. Treatment includes sleep and occupational therapy; music, art, and dancing; rites, rituals, and prayers to specific gods. Outcome depends on the will of the gods.

2000 BC   Mesopotamia: differentiation of treatment between physical and mental ailments. Physicians attempt to cast out evil spirits by calling on personal gods.

500 BC   Ancient Arabs, Greeks, and Romans: humane treatment, utilizing music, physical activity, good nutrition, music, and sedation with opiates.

460–377 BC   Hippocrates, Greek physician: isolates the brain as origin of thoughts and emotions; proposes natural, not supernatural, causes for mental disturbances; believes they can be treated. Advocate of humane treatment.

428–348 BC   Plato, Greek philosopher: advocates humane treatment. Psyche is the root cause of madness, a theory mirrored by modern Freudian theory.

384–322 BC   Aristotle, Greek philosopher: links the heart and mind; intelligence seated in the heart; mind regulates the heart. Integrates feelings, thoughts, and actions. Melancholia causes mental illness; music is the cure. Describes hereditary tendencies of mental illnesses.

372–287 BC   Theophrastus, Aristotle's student: describes up to thirty personality traits, foreshadowing modern concept of personality disorders.

25 BC–AD 50   Celsus, Roman author of *De Medicina*: wrath of the gods causes mental illness; whips, chains, starvation, and beatings are the cure.

AD 50–130   Aretaeus, Greek physician: views normal and abnormal behavior as a continuum; emotional disorders an exaggeration of existing personality traits. Observes both melancholia and mania can occur in the same individual. Predates Emil Kraepelin's nineteenth-century description of manic-depressive psychosis.

500–1500   Early and late Middle Ages: In Europe, fall of the Roman Empire saw rise of magic, witchcraft, superstition, and demonic possession, resulting in a long period of persecution, brutality, and torture. Mentally ill allowed their freedom if not deemed dangerous. Although some religious orders provide care, almost all caregiving establishments disappear. In Arabia, Muslims establish humane asylums and pursue Greek "scientific" approaches.

865–925   al-Razi (Rhazes), Persian physician: director of Baghdad hospital; establishes special section for the mentally ill, treating them with respect and understanding; contributes significantly to psychiatric ethics; uses primitive but dynamic form of psychotherapy.

1100   Mets, northern France: first record of asylum specifically for sufferers of mental diseases.

1247   London, England: Bethlem Royal Hospital established; accepts first "lunatic" patient in 1377. Refounded 1547 as St. Mary of Bethlehem specifically as insane asylum; becomes known as "Bedlam" (a corruption of the name); inmates become tourist attractions around the 1670s.

1407–1409   Valencia, Spain: first known establishment in Europe for mentally ill.

1492–1540   Juan Luis Vives, Spanish humanist: advocates Hippocratic principle for mental patients: "First do no harm." Witch hunts rampant.

1515–1547   Francois I, France: more than 100,000 mentally ill people killed during his reign.

1600–1800   Insane increasingly isolated from society and housed with vagrants, delinquents, and handicapped—usually in dungeons, often chained to walls. In Britain, private "madhouses" become prolific and profitable. Widespread attitude that insane behave like animals so should be treated as such; filthy, cruel living conditions predominate; cold-water immersion and mechanical devices to attempt cures. By late 1700s, some reform movements begin; emergence of psychology as a discipline.

1621 Robert Burton, English scholar and cleric: publishes *Anatomy of Melancholia*, noting specifically the role of traumatic loss in onset of melancholia.

1758 William Battie, English physician: pioneer in care and treatment of the insane; publishes *Treatise on Madness*, still in print. Supports therapeutic asylums and specially trained nurses.

1773 Williamsburg, Virginia: first North American insane asylum established.

1790s–1820s Philippe Pinel, France; William Tuke, England; Eli Todd, America: major reformers in treatment of mentally ill.

1812 Benjamin Rush, American physician: writes *Medical Inquiries and Observations upon the Diseases of the Mind*; earns him title of "Father of American Psychiatry."

1840s Dorothea Dix, American reformer: begins 40-year campaign to remove mentally ill from inhumane conditions in prisons; efforts result in establishment of thirty-two state hospitals for mentally ill over the next 40 years. On tour in mid-1800s, she convinces Pope Pius IX to investigate cruel treatment of Europe's mentally ill.

1840 U.S. census lists one category for mental illness: idiocy/insanity.

1844 American Psychiatric Association (APA) founded.

1850s Pierre Janet, French physician and psychologist; Sigmund Freud, Austrian neurologist and psychiatrist: pioneer scientific inquiry into human behavior.

1880 U.S. census lists seven categories of insanity: mania, melancholia, monomania, paresis, dementia, dipsomania, and epilepsy.

1892 American Psychological Association (APA) founded.

1895 Freud and Josef Breuer, Austrian neurologist: publish theories of the unconscious mind in *Studies of Hysteria*.

1899 Emil Kraepelin, German psychiatrist: distinguishes between schizophrenia and manic-depressive psychosis; defines mental decline at a young age as *dementia praecox*, eventually known as schizophrenia.

1900 Freud publishes *The Interpretation of Dreams*: "talking cures" developed; psychoanalytic era begins; psychotherapy becomes primary treatment for mental illness for several decades.

1906   Alois Alzheimer, German psychiatrist and Kraepelin's col-
league: announces his identification of abnormalities in a post-
mortem brain—senile plaques and neurofibrillary tangles—that
indicate Alzheimer's disease.

1908   Clifford Beers, United States: former mental institution
inmate publishes autobiography *A Mind That Found Itself*,
revealing his degrading and dehumanizing experience.
Establishes National Committee for Mental Hygiene, which
becomes National Mental Health Association, an advocacy
and education organization.

1913   John B. Watson, American psychologist: gives birth to behaviorist theory and concept of psychological conditioning.

1914–1919   Soldiers in World War I treated with talk therapy for newly
defined "shell shock," later known as post-traumatic stress
disorder (PTSD).

1929   Hans Berger, German psychiatrist: first person to image the
human brain. Using electroencephalograph (ECG), proves
the existence of electric potentials (voltage fluctuations).

1930s   Beginning of "golden age" of highly controversial insulin
coma and electroconvulsive therapies and frontal lobotomies for treating schizophrenia and other intractable mental
disorders.

1936   Egas Moniz, Portuguese physiologist: publishes his work on
frontal lobotomies.

1938   First human patient is given electroconvulsive therapy.

1920s–1940s   Asylums become mental hospitals; men and women become
trained nurses, with low pay and long hours. Asylums known
as "snake pits" after World War II due to overcrowding and
inadequate care.

1946   Harry Truman, U.S. president: signs National Mental Health
Act and calls for a National Institute of Mental Health (established 1949) to conduct research to reduce mental illness.

1949   John F. J. Cade, Australian psychiatrist: first to treat psychosis with lithium, still the mainstay for treating mania.

1950   Psychotropic drug therapy begins in earnest. Will fall far
short of the hoped for "miracle cure," but successfully allevi-
ates symptoms for hundreds of thousands.

1952   American Psychiatric Association publishes first *Diagnostic and Statistic Manual of Mental Disorders* (DSM).
DSM-IV-Text Revision published in 2000; DSM-V scheduled for 2011. Chlorpromazine (Thorazine) first used to
treat schizophrenia

1953 James Watson, American physicist, and Francis Crick, British physicist: unravel structure of DNA, beginning the era of genetic research.

1955 United States and Europe: numbers in psychiatric hospitals peak in mid-1950s

1959 R. D. Laing, Scottish psychiatrist: publishes *The Divided Self: An Existential Study of Sanity and Madness.*

1961 Thomas Szasz, American psychiatrist: publishes *The Myth of Mental Illness*; questions the very existence of mental illness. Strongly condemns coercive (forced) treatment.

1967 David Cooper, South African psychiatrist: coins the term "antipsychiatry"; antipsychiatry and other like organizations emerge, criticizing, challenging, and combating philosophies of mainstream psychiatry.

1970s Neuroimaging the brain becomes possible with noninvasive techniques. Massive deinstitutionalization begins, with subsequent increase in homelessness and incarceration of seriously mentally ill due to failure of community health system.

1979 Founding of National Alliance for the Mentally Ill, a consumer advocacy, support, and educational organization.

1988 MindFreedom Support Coalition International, a patient advocacy and survivor organization, established in United States. Managed care in mental health begins with Massachusetts instituting "carve-out" plans, contracting private insurance providers for mental health coverage.

1990s New-generation antipsychotics and antidepressants hit the market.

1993 Neuroimaging identifies three brain regions involved in schizophrenia.

1995 Through the U.S. military's psychopharmacology program, psychologists prescribe medication for the first time.

1996 First insurance parity law enacted; leaves loopholes allowing continuing insurance disparity between coverage of physical and mental illnesses.

1999 U.S. Surgeon General publishes landmark *Mental Health: A Report of the Surgeon General.*

2000 Researchers link the disrupted in schizophrenia 1 (*DISC-1*) gene to increased risk of schizophrenia.

2001 Robert Whitaker, American medical writer: publishes *Mad in America: Bad Science, Bad Medicine, and the Enduring Mistreatment of the Mentally Ill.*

2002   George W. Bush, U.S. president: forms New Freedom Commission on Mental Health, mandated to conduct in-depth study of mental health delivery services. New Mexico becomes first state to license psychologists to prescribe psychotropic medication.

2003   Researchers discover mutation in the G protein-coupled receptor kinase 3 (*GRK3*) gene in 10 percent of people with bipolar disorder.

2005   Researchers link a second gene—phosphodiesterase 4B (*PDE4B*)—to schizophrenia.

2006   Researchers discover first "risk" gene—fatty-acid transport (*FAT-1*)—specifically for bipolar disorder. Neither definitive causes nor cures yet found for mental illnesses. Stigma remains a major barrier to treatment and to general understanding of mental illness.

Glossary

5-HT 5-hydroxytryptamine (serotonin); a neurotransmitter found in the brain and other areas of the body; associated with mood, attention, emotions, and sleep. Low levels associated with depression

Acetylcholine a neurotransmitter in the somatic and parasympathetic nervous systems

Advocacy actively supporting or arguing in favor of something

Akathisia inner or motor restlessness; a feeling of muscular quivering, inability to be still; common side effect of neuroleptic drugs

Anticonvulsants drugs used to treat convulsions, such as in epilepsy, but often used to help control mania in bipolar disorder

Antidepressants medication used to alleviate depression

Antipsychiatry a philosophy that challenges the mainstream, biomedical model of psychiatry

Antipsychotics (neuroleptics) calming or sedating medication used to alleviate symptoms of psychotic episodes associated with schizophrenia and other disorders

Assisted outpatient treatment (AOT) involuntary outpatient commitment; court-ordered treatment, usually with medication, on an outpatient basis

Atypical antipsychotics newer (new-generation or second-generation) antipsychotics to treat psychotic episodes

Axon a long fiber on a nerve cell that carries the neuronal signal from that cell to others

Biological pertaining to the body of living organisms

Biomedical application of natural science (biology) to clinical medicine

Bodily humors Middle Ages concept of four bodily fluids (black bile, yellow bile, blood, and phlegm—each one associated with one of the four seasons, four basic elements of nature, and four bodily organs (gallbladder, spleen, liver, and brain/lungs, respectively)—thought to determine emotional and physical well-being

Capsulotomy one of four modern psychosurgical procedures, the others being cingulotomy, subcaudate tractotomy, and limbic leukotomy

Cell membrane thin tissue that covers the cell and regulates chemicals entering and exiting (stimulating) the cell

Central nervous system brain and spinal chord

Cingulotomy one of four modern psychosurgical procedures, the others being capsulotomy, subcaudate tractotomy, and limbic leukotomy

Coercive psychiatry Forced or involuntary treatment

Computed tomography (CT) a series of detailed, cross-sectional, computer-generated, X-ray images of the inside of the body

Concordance rates in genetics, the rate of occurrence of a particular trait in family members, particularly both twins

Copayment a fee determined by an insurance company that the insured individual pays for a particular health care service

Deductible amount an insured member must pay for eligible health services before the insurance company will contribute payments for such services

Dementia praecox irreversible mental decline before its time; at a young age

Dendrite a short fiber on a neuron that receives a signal from another neuron

Disclosure revealing something, such as information

Dopamine a neurotransmitter in the central nervous system

Dystonia abnormal muscle tone; neurologically activated involuntary and continuous muscle contractions

Ego in psychiatry, one of the three major divisions of the psyche, the others being the id and the superego, as opposed to common usage, which implies self-love or selfishness

Electroconvulsive therapy (ECT) passage of electrical currents through the brain to cause convulsions; used to treat severe depression and other intractable psychological disorders

Electroencephalograph (EEG) medical instrument to record electrical currents in the brain

Enzymes chemical substances (proteins) produced by living cells that cause certain chemical reactions

Exorcism a religious right or ritual to drive out evil spirits

Extrapyramidal side effects (EPS) the extrapyramidal system is a neuronal network in the brain involved in movement coordination; EPS are movement abnormalities caused by antipsychotic medications

GABA γ (gamma)-aminobutyric acid; an amino acid found in the central nervous system and the major inhibitory (restraining) neurotransmitter in the brain

Gene a segment of DNA involved in heredity

Genetics biological study of genes and their role in heredity

Glutamate a form of glutamic acid, an amino acid and one of the twenty essential building blocks of a protein

Guilty but mentally ill a legal plea or verdict in which an individual is guilty of a crime but also mentally ill

Hallucinations subjective sensations experienced by an individual with no presence of an appropriate stimulus or cause, which are yet perceived by the individual to be real

Human genome all genes on all human DNA

Hypomania a mood resembling mania but of lesser intensity

Id term coined by Sigmund Freud to describe the seat of primitive instincts and energies that underlie all psychic activity

Informed consent agreement by an individual to participate willingly in a contract after being informed of and understanding all risks involved

Inquisition a rigid and harsh tribunal once held by the Roman Catholic Church to suppress heresy

Involuntary commitment court-ordered commitment to a psychiatric hospital or ward against the individual's will

Libido emotional and psychic energy related to basic human instincts, particularly to sex drive

Limbic leukotomy one of four modern psychosurgical procedures, the others being capsulotomy, cingulotomy, and subacute tractotomy

Lobotomy an early, crude type of psychosurgery in which nerves in the front part of the brain were severed

Magnetic resonance imaging (MRI) noninvasive imaging technique; in imaging the brain, it allows reconstruction and visualization of brain images in all planes

Managed care an insurance method of managing medical expenses by controlling and limiting who provides care and what care is covered

Mania persistent abnormally elevated or expansive mood, often accompanied by hyperactivity, inflated self-esteem, severe insomnia, grandiose feelings, etc.

Medicaid a federally and state-funded health care program for the needy

Medicare a federally administered health care program for those over 65 years of age

Mental health parity equal insurance coverage for medical and psychiatric health services

Middle Ages historic period in European history between antiquity and the Italian Renaissance; generally considered to extend from the fall of the Roman Empire in the fifth century to the early fifteenth century

Monoamine oxidase inhibitors medication that inhibits the action of monoamine oxidase; used to alleviate depression and anxiety

Monoamine oxidase an enzyme in the cells of most tissues, including the brain, that affects the action of certain other neurotransmitters, such as serotonin and dopamine

Neuroimaging technological imaging of the brain

Neuroleptics (antipsychotics) drugs that reduce neuronal activity, with a tranquilizing effect

Neuron a nerve cell, usually with a body, an axon, and dendrites

Neurotransmitter a chemical substance that carries impulses, or messages, between neurons

New-generation antidepressants a new class of drugs, primarily selective serotonin reuptake inhibitors (SSRIs), which were developed in the 1990s to treat depression

Noradrenalin (norepinephrine) a hormone and neurotransmitter

Norepinephrine see noradrenalin

Not guilty by reason of insanity a plea or verdict in which the defendant is guilty of the crime but deemed so mentally incompetent at the time as to be unaware of or unable to understand the nature of the act or to control the behavior

Oedipus complex psychoanalytic theory developed by Sigmund Freud, in which a son unconsciously seeks sexual fulfillment with his mother

Paranoia delusions of persecution; unreasonable suspicion of others' motives

Parasympathetic nervous system originates in the brain stem and lower part of the spinal cord. Opposes physiological effects of the sympathetic nervous system: stimulates digestive secretions, slows the heart, constricts the pupils, dilates blood vessels

Parens patriae Latin for "parent of the country"; name of the legal doctrine by which the state has responsibility to care for those unable to care for themselves

Penis envy psychoanalytic theory developed by Sigmund Freud that psychological problems in some women and girls arise from a sense of being deprived of a penis

Phobia a powerful, irrational fear

Physiological functioning of living organisms

Positron emission tomography (PET) highly specialized, powerful, noninvasive technique for imaging the body's biological function

Postpartum period beginning after childbirth

Postsynaptic occurring after the synapse

Premium (insurance) amount an insurance company charges an individual to purchase a policy

Presynaptic occurring before the synapse

Protein any of a large group of nitrogenous organic compounds that are essential parts of all living cells

Psychiatry a medical specialty of diagnosis, treatment, and care of people with mental illnesses and of research into possible causes and treatment

Psychoanalysis a method developed by Sigmund Freud in which a psychiatrist or psychologist attempts to interpret a patient's expressed thoughts, emotions, dreams, etc., in an attempt to bring the unconscious into conscious awareness

Psychology scientific study of the human mind and mental states and of human and animal behavior

Psychosurgery an operation on certain areas of the brain in an attempt alleviate certain severe mental disorders

Psychotropic a substance that affects the mind, mood, or other mental processes

Reformation western European movement in the sixteenth-century, aimed at reforming some Roman Catholic Church practices and from which Protestant denominations evolved

Relativist proponent of relativism, a philosophical theory that truth and moral beliefs are not concrete but vary depending on who holds them

Selective serotonin reuptake inhibitors (SSRIs) drugs that prevent serotonin circulating in the brain from returning to the neuron that released it, thus allowing more serotonin to remain in the synapse; enhances mood and decreases depression

Serotonin see 5-HT

Single-photon-emission computed tomography (SPECT) noninvasive imaging technique that allows observation of the brain while it is functioning (thinking, responding to stimuli)

Somatic affecting the body rather than the mind

Stigma shame and disgrace attached to something, making it socially unacceptable

Subacute tractotomy one of four modern psychosurgical procedures, the others being cingulotomy, capsulotomy, and limbic leukotomy

Superego part of the mind, thought by Sigmund Freud to act as the ego's conscience, that develops through parental and societal moral standards and rules

Sympathetic nervous system sympathetic nerves originate inside the vertebral column near the center of the spinal cord; activates what is often termed the fight-or-flight response; increases heart rate, dilates pupils, constricts blood vessels, raises blood pressure

Synapse junction, or tiny gap, between two neurons

Talking cure early terminology for what later became known as psychoanalysis

Tardive dyskinesia involuntary muscle movements, often of the tongue and facial muscles; a common side effect of antipsychotic drugs

Thanatos Sigmund Freud's theory of the universal death instinct inherent in every individual

Trepanning drilling a small hole in the skull without damaging the brain

Vesicles tiny sacs at the end of axons that contain neurotransmitters

APPENDIX D

Further Reading

American Geriatrics Society. 1993, January 1. "Mental Health and the Elderly Position Statement." Available at http://www.americangeriatrics.org/products/positionpapers/mentalhl.shtml.

American Psychological Association. "How Psychotherapy Helps People Recover from Depression." Available at APA Help Center Web site. http://www.apahelpcenter.org/articles/article.php?id=49. Accessed 6/28/2006.

Andreasen, Nancy C. 1997. "What Is Psychiatry?" *American Journal of Psychiatry* 154(5): 592. Available at http://ajp.psychiatryonline.org/cgi/reprint/154/5/591

Andreasen, Nancy C. 2001. *Brave New Brain: Conquering Mental Illness in the Era of the Genome.* New York: Oxford University Press.

Antipsychiatry Coalition Web site. Available at http://www.antipsychiatry.org. Accessed 6/28/2006.

APRIL: Adverse Psychiatric Reactions Information Link. "Information: Zyban (Bupropion, also Known as Wellbutrin). Available at APRIL: Adverse Psychiatric Reactions Information Link Web site. http://www.april.org.uk/pages/zyban.html. Accessed 6/28/2006.

Barondes, Samuel H. 2003. *Better than Prozac: Creating the Next Generation of Psychiatric Drugs.* New York: Oxford University Press.

Bassler, M., and S. O. Hoffmann. 1994. "Stationäre Psychotherapie bei Angststörungen. Ein Vergleich ihrer therapeutischen Wirksamkeit bei Patieten mit generalisierter Angststörung, Agoraphobie, und Panikstörung." [Inpatient Psychotherapy of Anxiety disorders—A Comparison of Therapeutic Effectiveness in Patients with Generalized Anxiety Disorder, Agoraphobia and Panic Disorder] *Psychotherapie, Psychosomatik, Medizinische Psychologie* 44(7): 217–225. Available at http://www.ncbi.nlm.nih.gov/entrez/query.fcgi?cmd=Retrieve&db=PubMed&list_uids=7938367&dopt=Abstract.

Baughman, Fred A., Jr., with Craig Harvey. 2006. The ADHD Fraud: How Psychiatry Makes "Patients" of Normal Children. Oxford: Trafford Publishing.

Bola, John R. 2005. "Medication-Free Research in Early Episode Schizophrenia: Evidence of Long-Term Harm?" *Schizophrenia Bulletin* 32(2): 288–296. Available at Schizophrenia Bulletin Web site. http://schizophreniabulletin. oxfordjournals.org/cgi/content/abstract/32/2/288.

Boseley, Sarah. 1999, September 4. "Revealed: The Danger of Taking Prozac." *Guardian*. Available at http://www.guardian.co.uk/Archive/Article/0,4273, 3898467,00.html.

Breggin, Peter R. 2001. *Talking Back to Ritalin, Revised : What Doctors Aren't Telling You about Stimulants and ADHD*. Cambridge, MA: Perseus.

Breggin, Peter. "Vital Information About Ritalin, Attention Deficit-Hyperactivity Disorder and the Politics Behind the ADHD/Ritalin Movement." Available at Breggin Web site. http://www.breggin.com/ritalinbkexcerpt.html. Accessed 6/28/2006. (Summarized from *Talking Back to Ritalin*.)

Breggin, Peter R. 2003/2004. "Suicidality, Violence and Mania Caused by Selective Serotonin Reuptake Inhibitors (SSRIs): A Review and Analysis." *International Journal of Risk and Safety in Medicine* 16: 31–49.

Brown, Alan S., and Ezra S. Susser. 1996. "Prenatal Risk Factors in Schizophrenia." *Psychiatric Times* XIII(1). Available at http://www.psychiatrictimes.com/ p960121.html.

Carey, Benedict. 2006, March 21. "Revisiting Schizophrenia: Are Drugs Always Needed?" *New York Times*, p. F1.

Chen, Michelle. 2005, April 15. "Law to Force Mental Illness Treatment Raises Ire of Civil Libertarians." Available at New Standard Web site. http:// newstandardnews.net/content/index.cfm/items/1693.

Chesser, E. 1968. *Why Suicide?* London: Arrow.

Citizens Commission on Human Rights International. 2002, November 13. "The Silent Death of America's Children." Available at Citizens Commission on Human Rights International Web site. http://www.cchr.org/files/10582/death.pdf.

Citizens Commission on Human Rights International. "Involuntary Commitment: In Defense of Victor Gyory." Available at Citizens Commission on Human Rights International Web site. http://h11.protectedsite.net/index.cfm/6575. Accessed 6/28/2006.

Citizens Commission on Human Rights International. "Report on the Escalating Warnings on Psychiatric Drugs." Available at Citizens Commission on Human Rights International Web site. http://www.cchr.com/files/8011/ drug_report.pdf. Accessed 6/28/2006.

Citizens Commission on Human Rights International. "Violent and Lethal Restraints." Available at Citizens Commission on Human Rights International Web site. http://www.cchr.com/index.cfm/6689. Accessed 6/28/2006.

Coalition on Human Needs. 2005, August 30. "More People in Poverty, More Uninsured, in 2004." Available at Coalition on Human Needs Web site. http://www.chn.org/issues/statistics/povertyday.html.

Cohen, David, and Keith Hoeller. 2002, July 8. "Mental Health Insurance Parity Is an Empty Notion." *Los Angeles Times*, p. B11. Available at Alliance for

Human Research Project Web site. http://www.ahrp.org/AHRPinNews/ LATimes070802.php.

Crowley, Mary. 2003, October 1. "Better than Prozac: An Evening with Samuel Barondes." Available at New York Academy of Sciences Web site. http:// www.nyas.org/publications/readersReport.asp?articleID=8.

Darton, Catherine. 1999, February. "Notes on the History of Mental Health Care." Available at http://www.mind.org.uk/Information/Factsheets/History+ of+mental+health/Notes+on+the+History+of+Mental+Health+Care.htm.

Delate, Thomas, Alan J. Gelenberg, Valarie A. Simmons, Brenda R. Motheral. 2004, April. "Trends in the Use of Antidepressants in a National Sample of Commercially Insured Pediatric Patients, 1998 to 2002." *Psychiatric Services* 55: 387–391. Available at http://ps.psychiatryonline.org/cgi/content/ abstract/55/4/387?ijkey=3399dada35424e8e19158931b91d276f0038b9b0& keytype2=tf_ipsecsha.

Depression Guideline Panel. 1993, April. *Depression in Primary Care: Volume 2. Treatment of Major Depression. Clinical Practice Guideline Number 5.* Rockville, MD. U.S. Department of Health and Human Services, Public Health Service, Agency for Health Care Policy and Research. AHCPR Publication No. 93-0550. Available at Internet Mental Health Web site. http://www.mentalhealth.com/bookah/p44-d2a.html#Head1.

DeRubeis, Robert J., and Steven D. Hollon. 2002, May 23. "Study Finds Cognitive Therapy at Least as Effective as Drugs in Long-Term Treatment of Severe Depression." Available at University of Pennsylvania Web site. http://www.upenn.edu/pennnews/article.php?id=185.

DeRubeis, Robert J., Steven D. Hollon, J. D. Amsterdam, et al. 2005. "Cognitive Therapy vs Medications in the Treatment of Moderate to Severe Depression." *Archives of General Psychiatry* 62: 409–416. Available at Archives of General Psychiatry Web site. http://archpsyc.ama-assn.org/cgi/content/ abstract/62/4/409.

Dineen, Tana. 1998. "Psychotherapy: Snake Oil of the 90s?" *SKEPTIC* Magazine 6(3): 54–63.

Dineen, Tana. 2002. Brochure: "Manufacturing Victims: What the Psychology Industry is Doing to People." Dr. Tana Dineen Web site. http://www.tanadineen. com/DOCUMENTS/2002Brochure-Front.pdf.

Dotinga, Randy. 2006, June 5. "Antipsychotic Drug Prescriptions for Kids Soaring." *HealthDaily News.* Available at MedicineNet.com Web site. http://www. medicinenet.com/script/main/art.asp?articlekey=62357.

Double, D. B., ed. 2006. *Critical Psychiatry: The Limits of Madness.* New York: Palgrave Macmillan.

Eastgate, Jan. 2004. "Elderly Abuse. Cruel Mental Health Programs: Report and Recommendation on Psychiatry Abusing Seniors." Available at Mental Health Abuse: Exposing the Crimes of Mental Health Practitioners Web site. http://www.mental-health-abuse.org/elderlyAbuse.html.

Eells, Tracy D. 2000. "Psychotherapy of Schizophrenia." *Journal of Psychotherapy Practice and Research* 9: 250–254. Available at http://jppr.psychiatryonline.org/cgi/content/full/9/4/250.

Executive Order no. 13,263, *President's New Freedom Commission on Mental Health*, April 29, 2002. Available at White House Web site. http://www.whitehouse.gov/news/releases/2002/04/20020429-2.html.

Express Scripts. 2004, April 2. "Preschoolers Lead Growth of Antidepressant Use, Study Reveals." Available at http://phx.corporate-ir.net/phoenix.zhtml?c=69641&p=irol-newsArticle&ID=511187&highlight=.

Federwisch, Anne. 1997, December 11. "Mental Health Coverage in a Time of Managed Care." Available at NurseWeek Web site. http://www.nurseweek.com/features/97-12/mental1.html.

Frontline. 2002, October 17. "A Crime of Insanity: From Daniel M'Naughten to John Hinckley: A Brief History of the Insanity Defense." Available at PBS Web site. http://www.pbs.org/wgbh/pages/frontline/shows/crime/trial/history.html.

Garnett, Leah R. 2000, May 7. "Prozac Revisited: As Drugs Get Remade, Concerns About Suicides Resurface." *Boston Globe.* Available at National Association for Rights Protection and Advocacy Web site. http://www.narpa.org/prozac.revisited.htm.

Gilles-Thomas, David. 1989. "Lecture Notes for a Course in Abnormal Psychology: Mental Illness and Mouse Traps." Available at University of Buffalo Web site. http://ub-counseling.buffalo.edu/Abpsy/.

Glenmullen, Joseph. 2000. *Prozac Backlash*: *Overcoming the Dangers of Prozac, Zoloft, Paxil, and Other Antidepressants with Safe, Effective Alternatives.* New York: Simon & Schuster.

Goenjian A. K., D. Walling, A. M. Steinberg, et al. 2005. "A Prospective Study of Posttraumatic Stress and Depressive Reactions Among Treated and Untreated Adolescents 5 Years After a Catastrophic Disaster." *American Journal of Psychiatry* 162(12): 2302–2308. Available at http:// www.ncbi.nlm.nih.gov/entrez/query.fcgi?cmd=Retrieve&db=PubMed&list_uids=16330594&dopt=Abstract.

Hall, Carl T. 1999, September 15. "Big Rise Forecast in Mental Illness among Elderly." *San Francisco Chronicle.* Available at SFGate Web site. http://www.sfgate.com/cgi-bin/article.cgi?file=/chronicle/archive/1999/09/15/MN57728.DTL.

HayGroup. 1999, April. "Health Care Plan Design and Cost Trends—1998 through 1998." Available at National Association of Psychiatric Health Systems Web site. http://www.naphs.org/news/hay99/hay99toc.html.

HealthyPlace.com. 2002. "Depression in Elderly." Available at HealthyPlace.com Web site. http://www.healthyplace.com/communities/depression/elderly.asp.

HealthyPlace.com. 2002, March 12. "Medications for Treating Anxiety." Available at HealthyPlace.com Web site. http://www.healthyplace.com/Communities/Anxiety/treatment/medications_2.asp.

Human Rights News. 2003, October 22. "United States: Mentally Ill Mistreated in Prison. More Mentally Ill in Prison Than in Mental Hospitals." Available at Human Rights Watch Web site. http://hrw.org/english/docs/ 2003/10/22/ usdom6472.htm.

Jackson, Grace. 2005. *Rethinking Psychiatric Drugs: A Guide to Informed Consent.* Bloomington, IN: AuthorHouse.

Jamison, Kay Redfield. 2000. *Night Falls Fast: Understanding Suicide.* New York: Random House.

Jarrett, Robin B., Martin Schaffer, Donald McIntyre, et al. 1999. "Treatment of Atypical Depression with Cognitive Therapy or Phenelzine." *Archives of General Psychiatry* 56(5): 431–437. Available at Doctor's Guide Web site. http://www.pslgroup.com/dg/fdb32.htm.

Jeste, Dilip V., George S. Alexopoulos, Stephen J. Bartels, et al. 1999. "Consensus Statement on the Upcoming Crisis in Geriatric Mental Health: Research Agenda for the Next 2 Decades." *Archives of General Psychiatry* 56: 848–853.

Kessler, Ronald C., Patricia Berglund, Olga Demler, et al. 2005. "Lifetime Prevalence and Age-of-Onset Distributions of *DSM-IV* Disorders in the National Comorbidity Survey Replication." *Archives of General Psychiatry* 62: 593–602.

Law Offices of James Sokolove. *Paxil Withdrawal.* Available at Paxil Side Effects Law Suit Web site. http://www.paxil-side-effects-lawsuits.com/pages/ withdrawals.html. Accessed 6/28/2006.

Lenzer, Jeanne. 2005. "FDA to Review 'Missing' Drug Company Documents." *British Medical Journal* 330: 7. Available at http://bmj.bmjjournals.com/ cgi/content/full/330/7481/7.

Leucht, S., K. Wahlbeck, J. Hamman, and W. Kissling. 2003. "New Generation Antipsychotics versus Low-Potency Conventional Antipsychotics: A Systematic Review and Meta-Analysis." *Lancet* 361(9369): 1581–1589. Available at http://www.ncbi.nlm.nih.gov/entrez/query.fcgi?cmd=Retrieve&db= PubMed&list_uids=12747876&dopt=Abstract.

Levin, Aaron. 2005. "People with Mental Illness More Often Crime Victims." *Psychiatric News* 40(17): 16. Available at Psychiatric News Web site. http://pn.psychiatryonline.org/cgi/content/full/40/17/16.

Levine, Bruce. 2001. *Common Sense Rebellion: Debunking Psychiatry, Confronting Psychiatry—An A to Z Guide to Rehumanizing Our Lives.* New York: Continuum.

Mashour, George A., Erin E. Walker, and Robert L. Martuza. 2005. "Psychosurgery: Past, Present and Future." *Brain Research Reviews* 48: 409–419. Available at http://dura.stanford.edu/Articles/Psychosurgery.pdf.

Maxmen, Jerrold S. 1985. *The New Psychiatry.* Morrow: New York.

Mental Disability Rights International (MDRI) Web Site. http://www.mdri.org. Accessed 6/28/2006.

Mental Health Abuse. 2004. "Elderly Abuse. Cruel Mental Health Programs. Report and Recommendations on Psychiatry Abusing Seniors." Available at Mental Health Abuse Web site. http://www.mental-health-abuse.org/elderlyAbuse.html.

Mental Health Association of Alabama. "About Mental Illness." Mental Health Association of Alabama Web site. http://www.mhaca.com/about.htm. Accessed 6/28/2006.

Mental Health Works. "Mental Health Facts: Stigma and Mental Illness." Mental Health Works Web site. http://www.mentalhealthworks.ca/facts/sheets/stigma.asp. Accessed 6/28/2006.

Milane, Michael S., Marc A. Suchard, Ma-Li Wong, Julio Licinio. 2006, June. "Modeling of the Temporal Patterns of Fluoxetine Prescriptions and Suicide Rates in the United States." *PLoS Medicine* 3(6). Available at Public Library of Science Web site. http://medicine.plosjournals.org/perlserv?request=get-document&doi=10.1371/journal.pmed.0030190.

Mondimore, Francis Mark. 1999. *Bipolar Disorder: A Guide for Patients and Families*. Baltimore, MD: Johns Hopkins University Press.

Mosher, Loren. 1999, September/October. "Are Psychiatrists Betraying Their Patients?" Available at Psychology Today Web site. http://www.psychologytoday.com/articles/pto-19990901-000035.html.

Murphy, Gardner, and Joseph K. Kovach. 1972. *Historical Introduction to Modern Psychology*, 3rd ed. New York: Harcourt, Brace, Jovanovich.

Murray, Christopher J. L., and Alan D. Lopez. 1996. *The Global Burden of Disease: A Comprehensive Assessment of Mortality and Disability from Diseases, Injuries, and Risk Factors in 1990 and Projected to 2020.* Cambridge, MA: Harvard School of Public Health. (On behalf of the World Health Organization and the World Bank; distributed by Harvard University Press.)

National Alliance on Mental Illness. "Where We Stand: Confidentiality and Access to Medical Records." Available at National Alliance on Mental Illness Web site. http://www.nami.org/Content/ContentGroups/Policy/WhereWeStand/Confidentiality_and_Access_to_Medical_Records_-_WHERE_WE_STAND.htm. Accessed 6/28/2006.

National Alliance on Mental Illness. 2003, May. "About Mental Illness: Post-Traumatic Stress Disorder." Available at National Alliance on Mental Illness Web site. http://www.nami.org/Template.cfm?Section=By_Illness&Template=/TaggedPage/ TaggedPageDisplay.cfm&TPLID=54&ContentID= 23045.

National Alliance on Mental Illness. 2003, May. "Major Depression." Available at National Alliance on Mental Illness Web site. http://www.nami.org/Content/ContentGroups/Helpline1/Major_Depression.htm.

National Alliance on Mental Illness. 2005. "About Mental Illness." Available at National Alliance on Mental Illness Web site. http://www.nami.org/Content/NavigationMenu/Inform_Yourself/About_Mental_Illness/About_Mental_Illness.htm.

National Alliance on Mental Illness. 2005, April 1. "Senators Press for Funding Mental Illness Criminal Justice Programs." Available at National Alliance on Mental Illness Web site. http://www.nami.org/Content/ContentGroups/E-News/20052/April_2005/Senators_Press_for_Funding_Mental_Illness_Criminal_Justice_Programs.htm.

National Association for Rights Protection and Advocacy Web site. http://www.narpa.org/. Accessed 6/28/2006.

National Conference of State Legislatures. 2006. "Managed Care." Available at National Conference of State Legislatures Web site. http://www.ncsl.org/programs/health/managed.htm.

National Institute of Mental Health. 2000. "Depression." Available at National Institute of Mental Health Web site. http://www.nimh.nih.gov/publicat/depression.cfm#ptdep1.

National Institute of Mental Health. 2002. "Medications." Available at National Institute of Mental Health Web site. http://www.nimh.nih.gov/publicat/medicate.cfm#ptdep4.

National Institute of Mental Health. 2005. "Depression: What Every Woman Should Know." Available at National Institute of Mental Health Web site. http://www.nimh.nih.gov/publicat/depwomenknows.cfm.

National Institute of Mental Health. 2006. "The Numbers Count: Mental Disorders in America." Available at National Institute of Mental Health Web site. http://www.nimh.nih.gov/publicat/numbers.cfm.

National Institute of Neurological Disorders and Stroke. 2006, August 7. "Dementia: Hope Through Research." Available at National Institute of Neurological Disorders and Stroke Web site. http://www.ninds.nih.gov/disorders/dementias/detail_dementia.htm.

National Mental Health Association. "Electroconvulsive Therapy (ECT)." Available at National Mental Health Association Web site. http://www.nmha.org/infoctr/factsheets/ect.cfm. Accessed 6/28/2006.

National Mental Health Association. "Why Mental Health Parity Makes Economic Sense: Without Parity, We Waste Money." Available at National Mental Health Association Web site. http://www.nmha.org/state/parity/parity_economy.cfm#_edn15.

National Mental Health Association. 2000, March. "Depression: Depression in Women." Available at National Mental Health Association Web site. http://www.nmha.org/infoctr/factsheets/23.cfm#_ednref2.

Norfolk and Waveney Mental Health Partnership NHS Trust. "Transmitters." Available at Norfolk and Waveney Mental Health Partnership NHS Trust Web site. http://www.nmhct.nhs.uk/pharmacy/moa-neur.htm. Accessed 6/28/2006.

Olfson, Mark, Carlos Blanco, Linxu Liu, et al. 2006. "National Trends in the Outpatient Treatment of Children and Adolescents with Antipsychotic Drugs." *Archives of General Psychiatry* 63: 679–685. Available at http://archpsyc.ama-assn.org/cgi/content/short/63/6/679.

Palmer, Ann. "20th Century History of the Treatment of Mental Illness: A Review." Available at http://intotem.buffnet.net/mhw/29ap.html. Accessed 6/28/2006.

Page, Dan. 2006, June 12. "New Study Suggests Antidepressants Save Lives; Findings Show U.S. Suicide Rate Drops as Prescriptions Rise." Available at UCLA News Web site. http://ww.newsroom.ucla.edu/page.asp?RelNum= 7115&menu=fullsearchresults.

Pesola, G. R., and J. Avasarala. 2002. "Bupropion Seizure Proportion among New-Onset Generalized Seizures and Drug Related Seizures Presenting to an Emergency Department." *Journal of Emergency Medicine* 22(3): 235–239. Available at http://www.ncbi.nlm.nih.gov/entrez/query.fcgi?cmd=Retrieve& db=PubMed&list_uids=11932084&dopt=Abstract.

Philadelphia Association Home Page. http://www.philadelphia-association.co.uk/. Accessed 6/28/2006.

Porter, Roy. 2002. *Madness: Brief History*. New York: Oxford University Press.

Pringle, Evelyn. 2006, April 7. "Kids on ADHD Drugs: A Dangerous Path to Addiction." Available at Online Journal Web site. http://www.onlinejournal. com/artman/publish/article_672.shtml.

Pringle, Evelyn. 2006, April 25. "Drip Drip Drip—Paxil Info Leaks Out." Available at Lawyers and Settlements Web site. http://www.lawyersandsettlements. com/articles/paxil.html.

Prudic, J., M. Olfson, S. C. Marcus, et al. 2004. "How Effective Is ECT in Real Life?" *Biological Psychiatry* 55(3): 301–312.

Psi Cafe: A Psychology Resource Site. 2005, April 10. Biography: "John B. Watson: 1870–1958." Available at http://www.psy.pdx.edu/PsiCafe/KeyTheorists/ Watson.htm.

Psychnet-UK. 2003, July 20. "Disorder Information Sheet: Major Depressive Episode." Available at Psychnet-UK Web site. http://www.psychnet-uk.com/ dsm_iv/major_depression.htm.

RAND Corporation. 2000. "Does Involuntary Outpatient Treatment Work?" Law & Health Research Brief. Available at RAND Corporation Web site. http://www.rand.org/pubs/research_briefs/RB4537/index1.html.

Rheinstein, Bruce. 2000, March/April. "True Parity Means Eliminating Medicaid's IMD Exclusion." *Catalyst* 2(2). Available at Treatment Advocacy Center Web site. http://www.psychlaws.org/HospitalClosure/Rheinstein.htm.

Rhoten, Roger D. 2002, April 14. "Selective Serotonin Reuptake Inhibitors: A Critical Look at the Antidepressants and an Assessment of Potential Liability Faced by Their Manufacturers." Available at LEDA at the Harvard Law School Web site. http://lcda.law.harvard.edu/leda/data/446/Rhoten.html#fn242.

Ringbäck Weitoft, G., and M. Rosén. 2005. "Is Perceived Nervousness and Anxiety a Predictor of Premature Mortality and Severe Morbidity? A Longitudinal Follow Up of the Swedish Survey of Living Conditions." *Journal of Epidemiology and Community Health* 59: 794–798. Available at http://jech.bmjjournals.com/cgi/content/abstract/59/9/794.

Rose, Diana, Pete Fleischmann, Til Wykes, et al. 2003. "Patients' Perspectives on Electroconvulsive Therapy: Systematic Review." *British Medical Journal* 326: 1363. Available at http://bmj.bmjjournals.com/cgi/content/full/326/ 7403/1363.

Rothke, Joy. 1999, April 6. "Therapy Is All Talk." Interview with Ethan Watters. Available at salon.com Web site. http://www.salon.com/health/books/1999/ 04/06/therapys_delusions/print.html.

Saleem, Haneefa T. 2003, September 22. "New Law Moves Insurance Plans Closer to Total Mental Health Parity." U.S. Department of Labor Statistics. Available at Bureau of Labor Statistics Web site. http://www.bls.gov/opub/ cwc/print/cm20030909ar01p1.htm.

Sass, Kurt Douglas. 2002, April/May. "Hey Media, It's Our Turn." *New York City Voices.* Available at http://www.newyorkcityvoices.org/2002aprmay/ 20020517.html.

Schaler, Jeffrey A., ed. 2004. *Szasz Under Fire: A Psychiatric Abolitionist Faces His Critics.* Chicago, Open Court.

Schaler, Jeffrey A. 2005, August 28. "A Dialogue Between Vastal Thakkar and Jeffrey Schaler." Available at the Szasz Blog Web site. http://theszaszblog. blogspot.com/2005_08_01_theszaszblog_archive.html.

Schanche, Don, Jr. 2002, January 28. "Mental Illness History Comes Full Circle: 161 Years After Dorothea Dix Pulled Mentally Ill out of U.S. Jails, They Are Back Again." *Macon Telegraph.* Available at Treatment Advocacy Center Web site. http://www.psychlaws.org/GeneralResources/ article155.htm.

Schizophrenia.com. "Schizophrenia Facts and Statistics." Available at schizophrenia.com Web site. http://www.schizophrenia.com/szfacts.htm. Accessed 6/28/2006.

Science*Daily.* 2005, February 3. "More Homeless Mentally Ill Than Expected According to UCSD Study: Interventions Urged." Available at Science*Daily* Web site. http://www.sciencedaily.com/releases/2005/02/050201101738.htm.

Seligman, Katherine. 2002, March 17. "The Insanity Defense. Insanity Plea Debate Fanned by Yates Case. Courts' Standard Nearly Impossible to Meet, Experts Say." *San Francisco Chronicle.* Available at SFGate.com Web site. http://www.sfgate.com/cgi-bin/article.cgi?file=/chronicle/archive/2002/03/17/ MN144633.DTL.

Siebert, C. F., and J. F. Thogmartin. 2000. "Restraint-Related Fatalities in Mental Health Facilities: Report of Two Cases." *American Journal of Forensic Medicine and Pathology: Official Publication of the National Association of Medical Examiners* 21(3): 210–212.

Spitz, Deborah. 2003, August 11. "Guest Editor's Column: What Is the Role of Psychotherapy in Bipolar Disorder?—Part I." Available at Medscape Psychiatry and Mental Health Web site. http://www.medscape.com/viewarticle/459661.

Spitz, Deborah. 2003, September 20. "Guest Editor's Column: What Is the Role of Psychotherapy in Bipolar Disorder?—Part II." Available at Medscape Psychiatry and Mental Health Web site. http://www.medscape.com/viewarticle/ 462849.

State of Minnesota. Fourth Judicial District, District Court, County of Hennepin. Probate/Mental Health Division. 2002, August 20. "In the Matter of the Civil Commitment of: File No: P8-02-60415." Available at HealthyPlace.com Web site. http://www.healthyplace.com/Communities/Depression/ect/news/minnesotaforcedshock.asp.

Stavis, F. Paul. 1995, July 21. "Civil Commitment: Past, Present, and Future." *Quality of Care Newsletter.* New York State Commission on Quality of Care and Advocacy for Persons with Disabilities. Available at the Web site. http://www.cqc.state.ny.us/counsels_corner/cc64.htm.

Suicide Prevention Resource Center. "Suicide Prevention Basics." Available at Suicide Prevention Resource Center Web site. http://www.sprc.org/suicide_prev_basics/about_suicide.asp. Accessed 6/28/2006.

Swartz, Marvin S., and Jeffrey W. Swanson. 2004. "Involuntary Outpatient Commitment, Community Treatment Orders, and Assisted Outpatient Treatment. What's in the Data?" (Review Paper) *Canadian Journal of Psychiatry* 49: 585–591. Available at http://www.cpa-apc.org/publications/archives/CJP/2004/september/swartz.asp.

Szasz, Thomas Stephen. 1961. *The Myth of Mental Illness: Foundations of a Theory of Personal Conduct.* New York: Hoeber-Harper.

Szasz, Thomas Stephen. 1978. *The Myth of Psychotherapy: Mental Healing as Religion, Rhetoric, and Repression.* Garden City, NY: Achor Press.

Szasz, Thomas Stephen. 1998, March. *Thomas Szasz's Summary Statement and Manifesto.* Available at the Thomas S. Szasz, M.D. Cybercenter for Liberty and Responsibility Web site. http://www.szasz.com/manifesto.html.

Szasz, Thomas Stephen. 2004. *Faith in Freedom: Libertarian Principles and Psychiatric Practices.* New Brunswick: Transaction.

Timimi, Sami. 2005. *Naughty Boys: Anti-Social Behavior, ADHD, and the Role of Culture.* New York: Palgrave Macmillan.

Torrey, E. Fuller. 1972. *The Mind Game; Witchdoctors and Psychiatrists.* New York: Emmerson Hall.

Treatment Advocacy Center. 2003, January. "Suicide: One of the Consequences of Failing to Treat Severe Mental Illnesses." (Briefing Paper) Available at Treatment Advocacy Center Web site. http://www.psychlaws.org/BriefingPapers/BP6.htm.

Treatment Advocacy Center. 2003, October. "Violent Behavior: One of the Consequences of Failing to Treat Severe Mental Illness." (Briefing Paper) Available at Treatment Advocacy Center Web Site. http://www.psychlaws.org/BriefingPapers/BP8.htm.

Treatment Advocacy Center. 2005, March 30. "Assisted Outpatient Treatment: Results from New York's Kendra's Law." (Briefing Paper) Available at Treatment Advocacy Center Web site. http://www.psychlaws.org/BriefingPapers/BP18.pdf.

Treatment Advocacy Center. "Consequences of Non-Treatment." (Fact Sheet) Available at Treatment Advocacy Center Web site. http://www.psychlaws.org/GeneralResources/Fact1.htm. Accessed 6/28/2006.

Tulanelink.com. "Changing People's Minds, Tulane Style: A Tale from Two Perspectives." Available at Tulanelink.com Web site. http://www.tulanelink. com/tulanelink/twoviews_04a.htm. Accessed 6/28/2006.

U.S. Department of Health and Human Services. 2005. *National Expenditures for Mental Health Services and Substance Abuse Treatment 1991–2001.* United States Department of Health and Human Services Substance Abuse and Mental Health Services Administration. Available at the Web site http://www.samhsa.gov/spendingestimates/toc.aspx.

U.S. Public Health Service. 1999. *Mental Health: A Report of the Surgeon General.* United States Department of Health and Human Services. Available at the Web site http://www.surgeongeneral.gov/library/mentalhealth/ home. html.

Vives, Juan Luis. "Care of the Insane." Available at Humanistic Texts Web site. http://www.humanistictexts.org/vives.htm. Accessed 6/28/2006.

Wagner, Peter. 2002, April. "Incarceration Is Not an Answer to Mental Illness." *Mass Dissident.* Available at Prison Policy Initiative Web site. http://www. prisonpolicy.org/articles/massdissent040100.shtml.

Wang, Philip S., Sebastian Schneeweiss, Jerry Avorn, et al. 2005. "Risk of Death in Elderly Users of Conventional vs. Atypical Antipsychotic Medications." *New England Journal of Medicine* 353: 2335–2341. Available at http:// content.nejm.org/cgi/content/short/353/22/2335.

Watters, Ethan, and Richard Ofshe. 1999. *Therapy's Delusions: The Myth of the Unconscious and the Exploitation of Today's Walking Worried.* New York: Scribner.

Way, Bruce B. 1986. "The Use of Restraint and Seclusion in New York State Psychiatric Centers." *International Journal of Law and Psychiatry* 8(4): 383–393.

Weckowicz, Thaddeus E. 1984. *Models of Mental Illness: Systems and Theories of Abnormal Psychology.* Springfield, IL: C. C. Thomas.

Whitaker, Robert. 2002. *Mad In America: Bad Science, Bad Medicine, and the Enduring Mistreatment of the Mentally Ill.* Cambridge, MA: Perseus.

Williams, Rene. 2005, June 22. "WHO Urges Mental-Health Policy Review." Available at Science Daily Web site. http:www.medicineonline.com/conditions/ article.html?articleID=802&articleSource=12.

Winstead, Edward R. 2001, February 2. "Region of Chromosome 22 Linked to Bipolar Disorder, Again: Same Region May Contain Susceptibility Gene(s) for Schizophrenia." *Genome Network News.* Available at Web site http://www.genomenewsnetwork.org/articles/02_01/Bipolar_ disorder.shtml.

Wisconsin Coalition Against Sexual Assault. "People with Disabilities and Sexual Assault." Available at Wisconsin Coalition Against Sexual Assault Web site. http://www.wcasa.org/resources/factsheets/disabfact.html.

Wood, Derek. "What is Dementia?" Available at Mental Health Matters Web site. http://www.mental-health-matters.com/articles/article.php?artID=57.

Woody, G. E., A. T. McLellan, L. Luborsky, et al. 1989. "Severity of Psychiatric Symptoms as a Predictor of Benefits from Psychotherapy: The Veterans Administration-Penn Study." *American Journal of Psychiatry* 146(12): 1651.

Wooley C. F. 1982. "Jacob Mendez DaCosta: Medical Teacher, Clinician, and Clinical Investigator." *American Journal of Cardiology* 50(5): 1145–1148. Available at http://www.ncbi.nlm.nih.gov/entrez/query.fcgi?cmd=Retrieve& db=PubMed&list_uids=6753556&dopt=Abstract.

World Health Organization. 1999, September. *World Health Report 1999: The Growing Burden of Neuropsychiatric Disorders.* WHO Mental Health Bulletin No. 4. Available at WHO Web site. http://www.edifolini.com/edifolini/ whomsa.org/it/bulletin4_msa.html.

World Health Organization. 2005. *WHO Resource Book on Mental Health, Human Rights and Legislation.* Geneva, Switzerland: World Health Organization.

World Health Report 2001. "Mental Disorders Affect One in Four People." Press release, WHO/42, 28. Available at WHO Web site. http://www.who. int/whr/2001/media_centre/press_release/en/index.html.

World Medical Association. 2001. "The World Medical Association Resolution on the Abuse of Psychiatry." Available at World Medical Association Web site. http://www.wma.net/e/policy/a3.htm.

Wykes, T., P. Hayward, N. Thomas, et al. 2005. "What Are the Effects of Group Cognitive Behaviour Therapy for Voices? A Randomised Control Trial." *Schizophrenia Research* 77(2–3): 201–210. Available at http://www.ncbi. nlm.nih.gov/entrez/query.fcgi?cmd=Retrieve&db=pubmed&dopt=Abstract& list_uids=15885983.

Zuckoff, Mitchell. 2000, June 8. "Prozac Data Was Kept from Trial Suit Says." *Boston Globe.* Available at NARPA-National Association for Rights Protection and Advocacy Web site. http://www.narpa.org/prozac.data.suppressed.htm.

Zuvekas, S. H., J. S. Banthin, and T. M. Selden. 1998. "Mental Health Parity: What Are the Gaps in Coverage?" *Journal of Mental Health Policy and Economics* 1(3): 135–146.

ORGANIZATIONS AND WEB RESOURCES

Alzheimer's Association
World leader in Alzheimer research and support. First and largest voluntary health organization dedicated to finding prevention methods, treatments, and an eventual cure for Alzheimer's.
http://www.alz.org

American Psychiatric Association (APA)
APA is a medical association whose national and international member physicians work to ensure humane care and effective treatment for all persons with mental disorder.
http://www.psych.org

American Psychological Association (APA)

APA is a scientific and professional organization representing psychology in the
United States and is the largest association of psychologists worldwide.

http://www.apa.org

Anxiety Disorders Association of America (ADAA)

This is a nonprofit organization that promotes prevention, treatment, and cure of
anxiety disorders and improvement in the lives of all who suffer from them.

http://www.adaa.org

Bipolar World

The mission of this Web site is to provide information and a safe, interactive,
self-help environment for individuals with bipolar disorder to meet, share
with, and support each other.

http://www.bipolarworld.net

Breggin, Peter R., M.D.

Psychiatrist Peter Breggin has been informing the professions, the media, and the
public about the potential dangers of drugs, electroshock, psychosurgery,
involuntary treatment, and the biological theories of psychiatry for more than
three decades.

http://www.breggin.com

CHADD: Children and Adults with Attention Deficit/Hyperactivity Disorder

The nation's leading nonprofit organization serving individuals with ADHD and
their families, offering support for individuals, parents, teachers, professionals, and others.

http://www.chadd.org

Child and Adolescent Mental Health Fact Sheet

National Youth Violence Prevention Resource Center

Sponsored by the Centers for Disease Control and Prevention (CDC), this site is
a federal resource for professionals, parents, and youth working to prevent
violence committed by and against young people.

http://www.safeyouth.org

Citizens Commission on Human Rights International (CCHR)

CCHR, cofounded in 1969 by the Church of Scientology and Dr. Thomas Szasz,
investigates and exposes psychiatric violations of human rights. It has chapters
in thirty-four countries.

http://www.cchr.com

Depression and Bipolar Support Alliance (DBSA)

The nation's leading nonprofit, patient-directed organization, focusing on the
most prevalent mental illnesses—depression and bipolar disorder.

http://www.dbsalliance.org

HealthyPlace.com
The largest consumer mental health Web site, it provides comprehensive information on psychological disorders and psychiatric medications from both a
consumer and an expert point of view.
http://www.healthyplace.com

Human Rights Watch
This independent, nongovernmental organization is dedicated to protecting the
human rights of people throughout the world.
http://hrw.org

Judge David L. Bazelon Center for Mental Health Law
The mission of this leading legal advocacy organization is to protect and advance
the rights of adults and children who have mental disabilities.
http://www.bazelon.org

Mental Disability Rights International (MDRI)
An advocacy group, established in 1993, that is dedicated to promoting human
rights and full participation in society of people with mental disabilities
worldwide.
http://www.mdri.org

MindFreedom International
Unites one hundred grassroots groups and thousands of members in an effort to win
campaigns for human rights of people diagnosed with psychiatric disabilities.
http://www.mindfreedom.org

National Alliance for the Mentally Ill (NAMI)
NAMI, founded in 1979, is the nation's largest grassroots mental health organization
dedicated to improving the lives of persons living with serious mental illness
and that of their families.
http://www.nami.org

NARPA—National Association for Rights Protection and Advocacy
NARPA's mission is to empower those labeled as "mentally disabled" and to help
them learn to independently exercise their rights.
http://www.narpa.org

National Institute of Mental Health (NIMH)
One of twenty-seven components of the National Institutes of Health. Its mission
is to reduce the burden of mental illness and behavioral disorders through
research on mind, brain, and behavior.
http://www.nimh.nih.gov

National Mental Health Association (NMHA)
The nation's oldest and largest nonprofit mental health organization, it addresses
all aspects of mental health and mental illness through advocacy, education,
research, and service.
http://www.nmha.org

Schizophrenia.com

Started in 1995, Schizophrenia.com is a leading nonprofit Web community dedicated to providing high-quality information, support, and education to family members, caregivers, and individuals whose lives have been impacted by schizophrenia.

http://www.schizophrenia.com/about.html

Thomas Szasz Cybercenter for Liberty and Responsibility

Owned and maintained by psychiatrist Jeffrey A. Schaler. The intention of this site is to advance the debate about the psychiatrist and author of *The Myth of Mental Illness* Thomas S. Szasz's basic ideas and their practical implications.

http://www.szasz.com

Treatment Advocacy Center (TAC)

Founded in 1998, TAC is a national nonprofit organization working to eliminate legal and clinical barriers to timely and humane treatment for Americans with severe brain disorders who are not receiving appropriate medical care.

http://www.psychlaws.org

World Fellowship for Schizophrenia and Allied Disorders (WFSAD)

Established in 1982 in Canada, this is the only global organization dedicated to lightening the burden of schizophrenia and allied disorders for sufferers and their families.

http://www.world-schizophrenia.org

INDEX

Abuse, 101, 117
    depression, 39–40
    drugs, 136
    elderly, 143–144
    electroconvulsive therapy, 69,
        143–144
    insurance, 146, 154
    political: psychiatry, mentally ill,
        19–22, 97, 101, 117
    post-traumatic stress disorder, 45
    substance, 14, 17–18, 28, 30, 40,
        44, 53, 59, 109, 124, 145,
        152–153, 157
Addiction, 126, 155
ADHD. *See* Attention deficit
    hyperactivity disorder
Adler, Alfred, 51–52
Adolescents,
    depression, 40
    psychotherapy, 128
    psychotropic drugs, 81, 130, 134
Alzheimer, Alois, 13, 59
Alzheimer's disease. *See* Dementia
Antianxieties, 63, 64–65, 82–83
Anticonvulsants, 61–62, 75–76
Antidepressants, 62–64, 78–79, 133
    bupropion, 132
    children, 130, 132
    monoamine oxidase inhibitors
        (MAOIs), 63–64, 79–81, 125
    Prozac, 81, 130–132, 138–140
    selective serotonin reuptake
        inhibitors (SSRIs), 63–64,
        80–81, 130–132, 138–140

    tricyclics, 63, 79, 82
Antimanics, 61–64, 78
    lithium, 61–64, 73, 75–76
Antipsychiatry movement, 26, 90–91,
    95–97
Antipsychotics, 61–62, 76,
    132–133
    atypical, 77–78
    children, 133–134
    conventional, typical, 76–77
    elderly, 137
Anxiety disorders, 14, 26, 30, 39,
    42–46, 126
    generalized anxiety disorder
        (GAD), 43–44
    obsessive-compulsive disorder
        (OCD), 44
    panic disorder, 44
    post-traumatic stress disorder
        (PTSD), 45, 127
Assisted outpatient treatment (AOT).
    See Coercive psychiatry
Attention deficit hyperactivity
    disorder (ADHD), 129,
    134–136
Atypical. *See* Antipsychotics

Behavioral therapy, 54, 56–58, 127
    cognitive behavioral, 58–59
Biological causes, theories of, 7, 8,
    24–26, 38, 40, 59–60, 91, 93
Biomedical model, 26, 89–94
Bipolar disorder. *See* Mood disorders
Brain chemistry, 5, 53–54, 71–73, 86

ABOUT THE AUTHOR

MARIE L. THOMPSON is a writer and editor specializing in medical topics for reference works and medical journals.